GREAT SKIN

AT ANY AGE

GREAT SKIN
AT ANY AGE

HOW TO KEEP YOUR SKIN LOOKING YOUNG WITHOUT PLASTIC SURGERY

James H. Sternberg, M.D.
Thomas H. Sternberg, M.D.
and Paul Bernstein

St. Martin's Press ••• New York

Library of Congress Cataloging in Publication Data
Sternberg, James H.
    Great skin at any age.
    Includes index.
    1. Skin—Care and hygiene. 2. Beauty, Personal.
I. Sternberg, Thomas Hunter, 1908–   . II. Bern-
stein, Paul. III. Title.
RL87.S686   1982   616.5   82–17030
ISBN 0–312–34674–3

Design by Laura Hammond

10 9 8 7 6 5 4 3 2

Dedicated to my father

Thomas Hunter Sternberg, M.D.

*Professor Emeritus of
Medicine (Dermatology) UCLA Medical School*

JHS

Contents

Introduction

To most people, a "cosmetic procedure" means a face lift, a nose job, or a tummy tuck—that is, *surgery.* In the last decade, this surgery has come out into the open. There are many books on the subject. Celebrities talk openly about it. In fact, many people, rather than disappearing for a mysterious "vacation" and coming back "rejuvenated," actually brag about their surgery. They are *hurt* if friends fail to notice.

But, while cosmetic surgery can be successful and valuable under the right conditions, it is not for everyone. Some people develop keloidal scars. Others are prone to excessive bleeding. Others have the wrong skin type. Many are scared off by the cost—as much as $10,000 for the full treatment—and feel that going under the knife in a clinic or hospital is a bit drastic for the sake of looking more attractive.

In this book, we discuss all the ways of dealing with aging skin short of surgery. We will describe treatments for wrinkles that are not surgical, not expensive, take only a few minutes, and result in a noticeable, almost instantaneous improvement. We will also discuss how to delay the aging process of the skin and prevent wrinkling in the first place. We will also review the medical value of the pop beauty treatments for wrinkles—the result of our visits to some of the most prominent beauty salons in Beverly Hills.

Our goal is to answer all the questions you may have about basic care of the skin, specific problems of aging skin, beauty products such as soaps and cosmetics, home treatment plans, and medical office procedures. We will clear up many misunderstandings and debunk many myths. On the other hand, if we find a valid remedy in folk medicine or beauty magazines, we won't be afraid to say it works just because it wasn't on the curriculum in medical school.

The past few years have seen the advent of several new office procedures to treat the aging skin without surgery. We are very excited about Zyderm™ Collagen Implants, for instance, which use a natural substance found in the skin of all animals that can improve the appearance of scars, wrinkles, and frown lines. We were among seven hundred physicians involved in the testing of this product and now see it as a definite alternative to silicone injections.

5-Fluorouracil, a cream that seeks out and destroys damaged skin cells without affecting normal cells in any way and that leaves the skin looking softer, smoother, and more youthful, has revolutionized the treatment of aged skin due to ultraviolet light damage.

Our discussion of silicone, which has been a center of great controversy for several years for its use in breast augmentations and filling out facial wrinkles, will look into some of the horror stories and suggest how it can be used properly.

Among the other areas we will examine are:

• Freezing with liquid nitrogen to remove solar keratoses, warts, and sun spots (lentigines), a common and effective therapy.

• Electrodessication and curettage as an alternative treatment for solar keratoses, seborrheic keratoses, and certain types of skin cancer. (The procedure uses an electric needle to destroy the diseased area, scrapes off the damaged skin with a curette, and passes the needle lightly over the area once again to stop the bleeding.)

• Acid face peels for rejuvenating the skin, removing certain wrinkles or sun spots, and treating pigmentary problems. We include phenol, the deepest peel, and trichloroacetic acid (TCA).

• Proper hair care, including electrolysis, transplants, treatments for brittleness and breaking, and the truth about hair restorers, protein, and henna.

• Electric needle treatments for superficial blood vessels including spider angiomata, capillaries on the nose and cheeks, and veins in the legs.

• Saline injections for treatment of the fine superficial varicose veins that occur in the legs.

• Dermabrasion for wrinkles (especially around the mouth). A dermabrasion can be performed in the doctor's office under local anesthetic. It uses a wire brush or diamond fraise, spinning at a high speed, to remove the upper layers of skin. It has been used for many years, mostly for removal or improvement of acne scars, and replaces the older sanding technique.

The chapters fall into three general areas. First, we discuss the basic science needed to understand why the skin ages and why these treatments for it work. We've done our best to make it interesting, but let's not ask too much of Mother Nature.

Second, we discuss home skin care—what you can do for yourself, what you need to know about skin care products on the market, and how to keep your skin looking young no matter how many years have passed. We also look at the beauty salons, the cosmetics manufacturers, and what the beauty magazines have to say about care of the aging skin.

Third, we discuss the nonsurgical medical procedures

we just mentioned. We cover the procedures, complications, benefits, dangers, expectations, and recovery time. We give you all the information you will need to discuss the procedure intelligently with your physician and to choose which procedure, if any, is right for you. Because we write for a broad audience, we must make some general statements. But please remember that no two people are alike. People heal, pigment, and respond differently to injury, and have different susceptibility to allergies. For that reason, it is essential to find a physician you can trust and to discuss not only the procedures and how they apply to you, but your motives for undergoing the procedures and what you can realistically expect from them. Cosmetic procedures, just like anything in medicine, have their risks and their benefits. Only you, with a clear understanding of all possible results, can make the final decision.

How do you choose a physician? Our recommendation is that you talk with anyone you know, the family doctor, your pediatrician, or a friend of a friend. Ask them to recommend two or three physicians who perform the procedure you are interested in. Then make an appointment for a consultation with each of the physicians. Given three physicians of equal ability (and price and recommendation), go with the one you feel the most comfortable with. If you have no contacts at all, try the local medical school or medical association. Call the dermatology or plastic surgery department and ask for the names of three physicians who perform the procedure. It is important to have confidence in the person to whom you will entrust your appearance and your health.

Like any other profession, dermatology and cosmetic surgery is becoming more and more specialized. Since these nonsurgical procedures are often combined with plastic surgery for fine tuning, a brief discussion of the specialties is in order. General plastic surgeons operate on all parts of the body. Otolaryngologists do reconstructive and cosmetic surgery on the head and neck. Ophthalmologists may also do cosmetic surgery for the eyes. Dermatologists do skin sanding, hair transplants, and minor surgical procedures for skin lesions and may also perform cosmetic surgery on the face and eyelids. One good source of recommendations is the American Academy of Facial and Reconstructive Surgery, which has strict rules about training, experience, and competency. The Academy also offers a series of pamphlets of various aspects of plastic surgery and choosing a doctor, available for the price of a self-addressed envelope. You can write to them at 70 W. Hubbard Street, Chicago, IL 60610.

Just as patients look for good doctors, doctors look for good patients. It is essential that the doctor and patient establish open communication and that the patient have a realistic idea of what to expect—especially with a cosmetic procedure. A patient who does a lot of talking and no listening may not hear a word of the doctor's explanation. When the procedure is finished, that patient may be in for a big surprise—and blame it on the doctor.

The ideal patient has a realistic self-image, real cosmetic defects, and a realistic idea of what can and cannot be done about them. The ideal doctor realizes that what seems unimportant to him may, in fact, be of the utmost importance to the patient. Together, they work toward the best possible result. The doctor does not play up to the patient's ego with great promises of how life will change under his magic fingers; the patient does not play up to the doctor's ego, flattering him into attempting something he knows is ill-advised.

We live in a youth-oriented society. In many walks of life, success depends on a youthful appearance. We didn't make the rules, and we would change them if we could. But the fact remains that, for whatever reason, looking young is of great importance to many people. By understanding the fundamentals of skin care and the many medical procedures now available, we can keep the skin looking young even while the person inside grows old and wise. We all age. But not all of us need to *look* old.

GREAT SKIN

AT ANY AGE

ONE

Basic Facts About the Skin

The question "Why are there wrinkles?" is more often one of despair than scientific curiosity. If you think of yourself as a thirty-year-old but look in the mirror only to find a sixty-year-old staring back, it may be difficult to muster enthusiasm for the dictum, "You're only as old as you feel." If we are to deal with the treatment and delay of wrinkles, we must first understand the "why" of wrinkles.

Before you finish this book, you will most likely have absorbed more than you ever cared to about the effects of sun damage on the skin. The sun emits a full spectrum of wavelengths—from very short (invisible) through visible light to infrared (more readily appreciated as heat). We refer to the wavelengths that cause the most damage to human skin as the sunburn spectrum or UVB. Longer wavelengths, designated UVA, also cause the skin to age, but to a lesser degree. Ultraviolet light damage is *the* common denominator in the majority of skin changes we associate with age.

To understand why sun exposure damages the skin, we must first understand something about its makeup. The skin is composed of two layers of tissue—the epidermis, which is the outermost layer in direct contact with the environment, and the dermis, which lies directly beneath the epidermis. Supporting these is a subcutaneous layer made up mostly of fat cells.

The epidermis is a living, growing structure. It is multilayered and varies in thickness from one area of the body to another. Starting at the bottom or basal layer, cells divide, slowly migrating to the surface, changing from plump living cells into a thin, dry, resistant layer of intertwined, nonliving cells. This surface layer is called the *stratum corneum* and constitutes our barrier against nature. The cells of the stratum corneum ultimately disperse into the wind, down the drain, or, as the ads would have you believe, onto the shoulder of your blue suit.

In the epidermis reside the pigment-making cells that determine our skin color and cause us, given the appropriate stimulus, to tan. These cells, called melanocytes, account for one out of every ten cells in the basal layer.

The dermis, located below the basal layer of the epidermis, makes up most of the skin's mass. It contains the hair follicles, nerve endings, blood vessels, sweat glands, and oil glands, and varies in thickness from the scalp, where it is thinnest, to the back, where it is thickest. Collagen and elastic fibers make up a support network that gives the skin its tensile strength, limiting its ability to stretch, and its ability to snap back into its original shape, respectively. Loss of this resiliency characterizes certain pathological states. The ground substance, as far as we can determine, functions as a protective cushion for the other substances and provides them with nourishment and the basic elements necessary to their development.

At this point, we should explain what we do know

about how the sun and ultraviolet light rays can damage the skin. We know that UVL energy absorbed by the skin affects the DNA and RNA, the basic constituents of human cells, and that changes in these cells result in changes in the elastin, called solar elastosis and the collagen, called basophilic degeneration. Ultimately, these changes result in sagging, wrinkling, and a loss of support for the skin structures.

Sun damage does not occur in one day and patients of ours are often surprised to learn that sun damage has anything at all to do with the state of their skin. For some reason, these conversations always seem to take place on sunny days, when the same person who claims it has been years since he or she has done any sun bathing is usually wearing a short-sleeved shirt, no hat, and no protective sunscreen. One need not make an appointment with the sun or jet off to some exotic locale to get sun exposure; it is generally up there in the sky whether you are on the beach in Maui or on the freeway in Los Angeles with a bare arm hanging out the window. A bad sunburn today cannot make a wrinkle pop out tomorrow. Ultraviolet light damage is a cumulative process. It adds up over a lifetime until, eventually, the changes become noticeable. At that point, of course, the damage cannot be reversed.

As everyone knows, some people tan faster than others and some are more likely to burn than others. Skin type is hereditary. If your parents were fair-skinned, the chances are you are also fair-skinned; if they are dark, you are probably dark. We divide skin types into six categories:

Type 1: always burns when exposed to sun and does not tan.
Type 2: usually burns and tans only minimally.
Type 3: often burns and tans gradually.
Type 4: rarely burns and tans easily.
Type 5: never burns and always tans.

Type 6: black skin. (This is not meant to imply that a black
person cannot get a sunburn, only that it is hard to
notice. Black skin does get darker when exposed to the
sun.)

It might be assumed that people with darker skin have
more pigment cells, the melanocytes described earlier. But,
in fact, they do not have more melanocytes, just more and
larger melanosomes—the pigment—or melanin-containing
granules within the melanocyte, and these melanosomes are
more widely dispersed throughout the epidermis. The
melanosomes help protect the skin by absorbing and dis-
persing incoming ultraviolet light.

Tanning is a protective function, which is something of
a paradox since in order to get this protection we must accumulate ultraviolet light damage. A tan is *prima facie* evidence that the skin is accumulating sun damage. But the
fact that we are tanning also means that there are more pigment granules to absorb the ultraviolet light.

In addition to skin type, the intensity of the ultraviolet
light plays an important role in how much damage the skin
will accumulate. The intensity of the sun's rays varies with
the time of year, the time of day, the elevation above sea
level, and the latitude. If the sun's rays must travel a
longer distance through the atmosphere before reaching the
skin, they will be less intense. For that reason, it is often a
good idea to plan outdoor activities before 10 A.M. or after 2
P.M., when the sun is less intense. In fact, two-thirds of the
total ultraviolet light energy given off by the sun is during
this time span. Beware, too, of cloudy days. Yes, the atmosphere scatters and disperses the sunlight and less ultraviolet light reaches the skin's surface. But of the spectrum we
are concerned with, the ultraviolet sunburn spectrum, 70 to
80 percent will penetrate the clouds. Photochemical smog
(ozone), on the other hand, *will* filter out some of the ul-

traviolet light and is therefore protective, at least for the skin.

Beware of indirect sun exposure. The atmosphere scatters some of the sun's ultraviolet rays, which explains how one can get a sunburn even under an umbrella. Snow and sand reflect radiation.

Just how does this kind of sun damage manifest itself? The following list accounts for many of the factors usually associated with aging skin. Variations in skin thickness. Irregular pigmentation, either an increase or decrease. Increase in visible blood vessels such as the dilated capillaries *(spider telangiectasia),* often seen on the cheeks. Easy bruisability, most noticeable on the forearms. Cancer. Yellowish, often prominent discoloration. Brown "sun spots," most common on the backs of the hands and the face. Laxity, sagging, and wrinkles—that dreaded mark of aging.

Naturally, the areas that show most evidence of these changes are those most often exposed to the sun—the face, the hands, the area of the chest exposed by an open shirt. Men used to have more skin cancer on the ears and the back of the neck until they started letting their hair grow. Now the statistics are evening out, which shows that hair is a protection against the sun. Australia, a region of intense ultraviolet light populated mainly by fair-skinned Celtic immigrants, has the highest incidence of skin cancer in the world. Perhaps because of this dubious distinction they also have one of the better public education programs that stresses the importance of reducing sun exposure and detecting skin cancer. With ultraviolet light damage on the increase in our country, we would be wise to take similar steps to educate ourselves. As more of us spend more of our leisure time in tropical paradises, attired in next to nothing, we obviously expose ourselves to more sun.

Rather than reducing this exposure, some of us have taken artificial steps to prolong it. Indoor tanning centers have sprung up around the country offering, for a price of course, a choice of UVA or UVB artificial ultraviolet light irradiation. As we mentioned earlier, UVB is the more potent, cumulative, and permanent. But that does not mean that UVA-induced tan is without risk. Though you need a hundred times more UVA than UVB to get the same amount of redness, the risk of repeated exposures to UVA in doses large enough to tan is not known at this time. A recent bulletin of the American Academy of Dermatology's photobiology committee warned the public against tanning centers, saying they posed the same risks as any other source of ultraviolet light—skin damage and possibly skin cancer. For that reason, tanning for cosmetic purposes should not be considered a safe, innocuous procedure. In fact, there is only one case that might justify the use of tanning centers: a person living in a cold climate planning a winter vacation in a warm climate, who wants to prepare his paste-white skin in advance to avoid having it turn lobster-red and ruin his vacation. Others, particularly those with certain skin diseases that get worse when exposed to ultraviolet light, should have no use for tanning centers. (More information is available from a brochure entitled *A Word of Caution on Tanning Booths,* published by the Food and Drug Administration with the assistance of the American Academy of Dermatology's photobiology committee.)

To further suggest the extent to which we are overdoing the sun-god routine, we are now seeing greatly increased evidence of sun damage in young people. While it used to be very rare to find skin cancer in a thirty-year-old, and it is still not commonplace, we are seeing more and more of it—mostly in skiers and surfers. In both sports, the reflective properties of snow or sand add to the exposure. The sun cannot be escaped under water; ultraviolet light penetrates at least three feet. Recent data indicate that malignant melanoma, the most important of the skin cancers, is related to chronic exposure to ultraviolet light.

We do not want to leave you with the impression that the skin is completely defenseless. In fact, the skin has a few ways of fending off those UVL rays. First, the stratum corneum, that outermost layer of the epidermis, reflects a certain percentage of UVL. A bit more is dissipated by being absorbed in the skin, thanks to certain proteins in the cells of the epidermis. And, of course, the skin's pigmentation is the best defense. Not even the environment is totally against us. Window glass, for instance, filters out UVL in the sunburn spectrum—just compare the difference between the side of the body that is exposed to the open window in an automobile to the other side.

Nor do we mean to leave you with the impression that the sun is entirely a villain. Few things are entirely bad. Without the sun's full spectrum of visible light, life could not exist on this planet. The infrared spectrum provides our heat and UVL helps the skin produce Vitamin D. Older people whose skin has lost the ability to produce Vitamin D_3, an essential in preventing bone fractures, and are unable to replace it through their diets could make up the difference by exposure to the sun. Unfortunately, no one knows just how much sun exposure would be necessary to do that nor even what kind of sun is most conducive to Vitamin D production. Perhaps different skin types require different amounts of sun (a logical conclusion) and the amount could also be affected by the climate and latitude.

We should also not discount the psychological effect of the sun on the human psyche. Many patients tell us that the warm sun, especially near the ocean or a lake, has an immensely calming effect. This comes as no surprise, since we will freely confess to feeling better when the day is clear and sunny. The sun may be the cheapest known form of psychotherapy and, with adequate protection, it can be safely enjoyed.

Hormonal changes that accompany aging have results that are definitely noticeable. In hair, the most obvious is, of course, male pattern baldness, for which we have no acceptable treatment except transplants. After thirty, hair growth on the ears increases in men. Don't ask us what part this plays in nature's grand design. It is probably genetic and may even be carried on the Y chromosome. Women's hair may thin but they rarely go bald; it may be hereditary. Older women commonly develop gray, coarse hairs on the face, which is believed to be a result of hormonal changes, though the exact mechanism of graying hair is not understood. One theory credits a decrease in enzyme activity of melanocytes in the hair bulb, which is responsible for hair color. Hormones also cause pubic and axillary hair to thin.

Hormones are also responsible for a decrease in sweating—and you thought you were just getting calmer in your old age. Actually, sweat is very important as a moisturizer for the skin, providing four of man's natural moisturizers —lactic acid, urea, sodium chloride, and pyrrolidone. As the eccrine sweat glands, which are responsible for both nervous sweating and sweating that accompanies exercise, slow down, the skin may tend to dry out.

The oil or *sebaceous* glands, being primarily stimulated by androgens, the male hormones, behave differently in men than they do in women. In men, they are active until about eighty years of age. In women, androgen output (from the ovaries and adrenal glands) gradually decreases after menopause. The glands themselves get larger in women because turnover of cells slows down, but they produce less oil, thanks to the decrease in androgen output. Since the oil glands also help hold moisture in the skin, their *ritardando* can also contribute to the dry skin problem.

As the skin thins and production of oil and natural

moisturizers decreases, the skin dries and begins to itch. Dry skin is the most common cause of generalized itching or *pruritis*. Nerve endings, though fewer in number, are unfortunately no less sensitive. With age, it becomes easier and easier to trigger an itch-scratch cycle with external factors such as dry weather, the lower humidity of winter, clothing that rubs against the skin, certain soaps, steam heaters, and even boredom. (Dry skin is, however, not the only cause of pruritis; there are also internal causes that are beyond the scope of this book. The possibilities include drugs, internal malignancy, diabetes, hyperthyroid, liver or renal disease.)

QUESTIONS AND ANSWERS

Q. Why do I get these ugly purple spots on my arms and hands?

A. Chronic sun exposure decreases and damages the ground substance of the dermis, which can then no longer support and protect the blood vessels. The least trauma to the arms or hands leads to leakage of blood under the skin, which we call *purpura* and you call ugly. Many treatments have been tried, including Vitamin C, Vitamin E, and zinc, but we have yet to see anything work other than extreme caution. The spots will take care of themselves.

Q. Why is it that, now that I'm older, I seem to take so much longer to heal?

A. The rate of growth, or turnover rate, in the stratum corneum decreases with age. For example, a person over sixty-five takes 50 percent longer for blistered or abraded skin to re-epithelialize (as we call it) than does in a young adult.

Q. Is there any scientific rationale for facial massage?

A. Since it has been demonstrated that dermal blood vessels do decrease in number with age, gentle massage may in fact be of some value. Take it easy though, especially if your skin is sun-damaged. Over-manipulation could damage the underlying tissues.

Q. If wrinkles are a result of sun damage, as you say, why do most of us tend to get wrinkles in only one part of a damaged area?

A. Sun damage is not the *only* cause of wrinkles, just the principal one. Fine-line wrinkles may first result from the stress of repeatedly using the same facial muscle in one area—for example, the fine lines around the mouth from constantly puckering the lips or the frown and tension lines between the eyebrows from constantly frowning. As the underlying tissues accumulate sun damage, these points of stress turn into deeper permanent wrinkles.

Q. I've heard that smoking affects the skin. How does that happen?

A. A recent study of smokers found that, at age thirty, there was not much difference between the skin of smokers and nonsmokers but, by age forty or fifty, there was a very apparent difference. One explanation is that smokers use their facial muscles more, puckering their lips and squinting their eyes, and that this constant and continual stress causes the skin to age faster. Another explanation is that toxic substances in the smoke cause premature aging, but there are no studies to support this notion. Whatever the reason, the results are the same—premature wrinkles.

Q. Does working in an air-conditioned environment cause wrinkles?

A. Air conditioning reduces the relative humidity in a room and makes the air drier. When the relative humidity is below 30 percent, the skin gives up water to the air and becomes dehydrated, which accentuates existing fine lines and wrinkles. For treatment of this problem, we refer you to the chapter on home treatments and moisturizers.

Q. How can the sun be so dangerous when our ancestors spent their lives in it?

A. Rest assured, they got just as much sun damage and skin cancer as we do. It's just that they had more pressing concerns, like starvation, pestilence, and what to do about sabre-tooth tiger bites. A purse-string wrinkle was simply not the earth-shaking disaster it is today. Let's hear it for progress.

TWO

Delaying the Aging Process

We have no cure for aging. Although we would like to tell you how to prevent it, we cannot. Ponce de Leon spent years looking for the fountain of youth, and where is he today? Perhaps some day we will find the cure for aging, which will by definition be a potion for immortality, and if so, we would expect it to come with a lifetime guarantee. Until then it would be misleading to talk about preventing the aging process.

We can, however, tell you quite a bit about *delaying* the aging process, especially in the area where it most prominently manifests itself—on the skin. Because the skin is one of the body's major organs, we might expect it to age just as the other organs do. But there is one important difference. Your liver is hidden away inside somewhere, but your skin spends a lifetime being exposed to sun, wind, heat, cold, harsh soaps, detergents, dyes, perfumes, rough and chemically-treated clothing, chemicals of all sorts, and self-injury from rubbing, picking, and scratching. It's a wonder the skin lasts as long as it does.

If your skin looks old, it is often assumed that the rest of you is just as old. We take the skin for some kind of biological I.D. card, with "age" filled in indelibly. But not only is this I.D. card often in error, forging a new one is a relatively simple matter. The skin often lies terribly on the question of age, because it is so easy for the skin to age prematurely. Naturally, the skin ages; we would not deny that. But look at the skin under your bathing suit or on the insides of your arms. Why is that skin so light and firm, not much changed from the way it looked thirty years ago? Why does some of your skin look old, when you know that the rest of your body is young and healthy?

Environment is the difference, and the biggest single factor by far in the environment's damage to your skin is the sun. The sun's rays can burn the skin; they can produce damage by radiation; they can produce wrinkling; and they can produce skin cancer. This should not come as a great surprise, yet our beaches are still crowded by sunbathers deliberately building up a tan. The most important idea we can communicate in this chapter is that sun damage to the skin starts early in life, even though it may not manifest itself until one is forty or fifty years old. It is cumulative. And it is irreversible.

We have already discussed the skin's natural protective mechanisms. If you spent your life in a closet, that would be sufficient to keep your skin soft, smooth, and wrinkle-free for many years. Few people find that solution acceptable. They go to the other extreme, in fact, deliberately cultivating the bronzed look that our culture currently finds attractive. It *is* possible to get out in the sun, even to get a good tan, and not cause as much damage as we often do.

A good sunscreen is the next best thing to a closet for protecting the skin. By a sunscreen we mean, to slip into medical jargon for a moment, a topically applied chemical that protects the skin from ultraviolet light radiation. Sun-

screens have been available for many years over the counter
(that is, without a prescription), and a panel of the Food
and Drug Administration cited sunscreens, used regularly,
as an aid in preventing premature aging and the development of skin cancer. While we do agree, we should point out
that the FDA conclusion was based on animal studies and
there have been no long-term studies made in man. The animal studies are very convincing in the areas of tanning response, skin tumor development, and reduction of acute
sunburn. Studies in man on the difference in tanning and
burning with and without sunscreens have, as might be expected, shown sunscreens to be quite effective.

Most people think of sunscreens as a prevention
against acute sunburn, which of course they are. But since
long-term exposure to the sun's radiation causes the cumulative damage that results in wrinkles, skin cancer, skin
laxity, and the rest, it is perhaps time we started looking at
sunscreens as long-term protection. The sun's damage begins the very first time the skin is exposed and continues to
accumulate. If you are concerned with keeping this damage
to a minimum, we would recommend the use of a sunscreen
at all times. It should be part of your morning ritual.

What is the perfect sunscreen? It must be effective (obviously), inexpensive, and nonallergenic. It must reflect infrared rays, since ultraviolet damage is exacerbated by
heat. It should stay on with one application, not be removed
by a dip in the water, and it should not detract from one's
appearance or be inconvenient to use. That is our idea of
the perfect sunscreen—and it does not exist.

There are, however, some excellent products available
and even better ones on the horizon. A sunscreen generally
reduces the ability of ultraviolet light to penetrate the skin
in one of two ways: it can either reflect the light like a mirror or absorb it to keep it from penetrating. Some sunscreens contain both reflective and absorbing agents.

Reflective sunscreens, also called opaque sunscreens, block the full spectrum of ultraviolet light and thus give maximum protection. But they are very messy products and thus not too popular except with good-looking life-guards who smear the white, gooey stuff all over their noses —probably the only reason reflective sunscreens have gained any popularity at all. How a sunscreen looks is a legitimate consideration in getting people to use it. Most people find the taste of a lip balm mixed with a hamburger unappealing. While the reflectors have been accepted by surfers and skiers for use on the nose and lips, because they are so effective, no one really wants to use them on the whole body. Reflective sunscreens usually include zinc oxide, titanium dioxide, red veternery petroleum (RVP), or talc.

Of the absorbing sunscreens, the most popular—or at least the most widely used—is para-aminobenzoic acid and its esters, commonly known as PABA. Absorbing sun-screens usually come in three forms—a lotion, a cream, or a gel and absorb only the sunburn spectrum (UVB). Al-though the exact ingredients in many of these products are constantly changing, Presun® and Pabanol® usually con-tain pure PABA. Since these are currently classified as drugs rather than cosmetics, their ingredients must be in-cluded on the label. Thus, you can make sure they do con-tain PABA. If they contain other ingredients, check with the chart provided elsewhere in this chapter to see what rays those other ingredients block. PABA esters are gener-ally more likely to wash off than pure PABA, though some manufacturers would disagree. They do, however, absorb similarly; some examples of these products are Eclipse®, Sundown®, and Block-Out®.

While the absorbing sunscreens are very effective, they do have a few drawbacks. Liquid sunscreens have an alcohol base which, while acceptable for people with oily skin or acne, can be very uncomfortable for people with dry skin. People with sensitive skin conditions will often find that these products can sting. Since the liquids are clear, it is easy to miss parts of the skin when applying them. If these liquids (containing pure PABA) are spilled on clothing, they stain. They amply penetrate the outer layer of the skin, the stratum corneum, which delays their being washed off by swimming or sweating—but only if you apply them in advance, giving them time to do so. We recommend applying all sunscreens one hour before going out in the sun and again after swimming or perspiring. With cream-based products, the problems associated with alcohol obviously do not apply.

Other UVL absorbers include the cinnamates and benzophenones, contained in such products as Solbar®, Maxafil®, Uval®, and RV Paque®. Many substances contain both reflective and absorbing chemicals, giving a wider range of protection (both UVA and UVB). The salicylates and anthranilates, if used together, can block both UVA and UVB. Finally, the heavy cream-based sunscreens, especially those that combine reflective and absorbing sunscreens seem to have the most resistance to removal.

A new PABA-free sunscreen due to hit the market soon seems, from preproduction testing and information, to promise some new advantages. It will have a very high resistance to the sun (the highest to date), and, if the reports are correct, will not wash off. Because it will probably be marketed by several companies under several names, and as a lotion, a cream, or a clear liquid, we do not know exactly what to call it. Among the possible names it will be known by is Tiscreen®; but we recommend you consult your dermatologist for the latest information.

While on the subject of new products, we might mention the "quick suntan pills" now being sold over the counter in Canada and France. Since a suntan is a natural defense against the sun, might this be another way of gain-ing protection without damaging the skin? Unfortunately not because the product does not stimulate pigment increase, which is how the skin protects itself. It is a synthetic carotenoid, a substance that occurs naturally in vegetables and gives a distinctive orange/red hue that is easily recognized when taken orally and deposited in the fat tissues. You get a tan—if you call that a tan—but you don't get the tan's protection.

Before we lose you completely with this talk of staying out of the sun and screening out the rays, let us emphasize that it *is* quite possible to get an attractive tan while keeping skin damage to a minimum. Though the usual sunburn rays are in the 290–320 nanometer range, and this spectrum accounts for the lion's share of damage, the longer rays (up to 400 nanometers) can result in a safer tan, though it takes more time and energy. With the right combination of sunscreens, you can tan without burning.

A Sun Protective Factor (SPF) is now on the product label of sunscreens, which tells you, simply, how much protection they can offer. Different chemicals and different concentrations absorb different amounts of UVL. The SPF is based on something called the minimal erythema dose (MED), i.e. the least amount of UVL that will produce redness on the skin. If you normally get that first touch of redness in twenty minutes without a sunscreen, but it takes two hundred minutes with a certain sunscreen, you can calculate the SPF by dividing two hundred by twenty. Thus, the SPF for this particular sunscreen is ten. Calculating backward, if a sunscreen has an SPF of fifteen, that means that if you usually get red in ten minutes the sunscreen will allow you to go ten minutes multiplied by the SPF of fifteen before getting red—or one hundred fifty minutes.

We urge you to avoid tanning for the sake of tanning. However, we recognize that many of you will not heed that advice for whatever reason. Therefore, we offer our advice for getting that unadvised tan with minimal skin damage.

While getting your tan, use a sunscreen with an SPF of eight. It will take longer, but it will work. Once you are tan, switch to a sunscreen with an SPF of fifteen, which will allow you to maintain the tan. This procedure will not eliminate the ultraviolet light damage. It will reduce it. Also it helps to start off with small, measured increments of sun exposure, e.g. twenty minutes every day or every other day.

If the Food and Drug Administration continues its present policies with regard to classification of sunscreens, we can hope for more standardization and a more reliable SPF number. Those products sold to enhance tanning are considered cosmetics. But those sold to reduce sunburn are considered drugs, since they "prevent disease and/or affect the structure or function of a body system."

Everyone should consider using a lip sunscreen. Cold sores (strictly speaking, a herpes simplex infection of the lips) are often triggered by the sun. Certain types of skin cancer are more aggressive when they occur on the lips. Sun Stick,® R V Paba Stick®, Uval Sun® and Wind Stick®, and Chapstick® 15 are effective lip sunscreens.

If you have acne, there are certain sunscreens you should avoid. Anything containing cocoa butter, coconut oil, or petrolatum can aggravate acne and even cause a type of acne we call *acne cosmetica.* On the other hand, as we mentioned previously, alcohol-based sunscreens, with their drying properties, can be beneficial for acne.

If you want to continue to look as young as you can, we recommend making daily use of a sunscreen as much a part of your routine as brushing your teeth.

Sun damage is the primary cause of aging skin and thus protecting the skin from the sun is the best way to keep the skin looking youthful. We would, however, like to touch on a few other ways of delaying the aging process before we conclude this chapter.

We are often asked about internal treatments for the skin, especially vitamins and hormones. We can state categorically that neither vitamins nor hormones delay aging of the skin nor is of any cosmetic benefit. The only influence diet has on the skin's appearance is the general relationship of diet to good health and, hence, healthy skin.

Facial exercise or vigorous massage is sometimes promoted as a way of keeping the skin youthful, but in fact can have just the opposite result. The tension that exercise and massage create for the skin, especially with older or sun-damaged skin can increase the pre-existing damage.

Bland and unscented creams as needed for moisturizing are useful for lubricating dry skin and will be discussed in the chapter on home treatment. At this time, though, we should caution you against harsh and perfumed soaps which, combined with exposure to the sun, can in rare cases severely damage the skin.

Chronic irritation of the skin contributes to premature aging, as does self-inflicted damage such as picking and scratching. Picking and scratching can leave permanent scars and are habits worth breaking.

Frown lines on the forehead, between the eyes, and around the mouth, resulting from nervous tension, can become permanent with time due to the constant mechanical stress on the underlying tissue. If you find a foolproof way to eliminate stress, strain, and nervous tension, you can write your own book.

Hyperpigmentation, i.e. increase in color, can be produced by the interaction of UVL and certain perfumed creams and some internal medication. Most people are aware of the hyperpigmentation of pregnancy, called chloasma, but are not aware that it can also be produced by contraceptive pills. Any unusual pigmentation on the face should be examined by a physician.

The melanin that gives hair its color also has a protective function. Blonde or bleached hair is more vulnerable to the damaging effects of the sun than brown hair. Since hair is a dead structure, it has no means of repairing itself. Thus, the damage of sun exposure, harsh shampoos, dyes, bleaches, curling lotions, combing, and brushing is additive.

One does not ordinarily think of nails as victims of aging since nail polish can usually conceal any damage. But the nails, like all other tissues, do change with time—and for the worse. Nail changes associated with aging include drying of the nail plate, brittleness with cracking, and easy breaking of the nail tips with splitting and ridging. They also grow at a slower rate. In fact, the growth rate decreases by about 50 percent during a typical lifetime. Though hormones play a part in this, there are two other explanations. One, blood circulation to the nail matrix, that area behind the nail where it first starts to grow, decreases. Two, our old friend ultraviolet light has recently been fingered, so to speak, as the culprit. While no one will deny that brittleness is a result of aging, no one can say why. If you were born with brittle nails and have always had them, there is nothing that can be done. But if, as often occurs in females between the age of thirty-five and fifty, the nails are unusually brittle only on occasion, it may be the result of a thyroid disease. More often there is no disease. The brittleness just comes and goes and, again, no one knows why.

The best advice we can offer for coping with aging nails comes from Dr. Nia Terezakis of New Orleans, who places a premium on meticulous nail care and avoiding severe cracking, peeling, and chipping. Her advice? Finger pads to protect the fingertips, cotton gloves for everyday chores, and buffing to remove loose nail debris and smooth the nail plate. We can add a suggestion of our own. Soak the nails in water for five minutes. Then remove them and soak them in warm—*not* hot—oil for five minutes. Liquid petrolatum, olive oil, or a bath oil is fine for this purpose. After the oil, rub a little moisturizer into the nail bed, to lubricate and increase the circulation to the finger and, thus, to the nail matrix. 100 mg of niacin daily has been recently recommended for brittle nails. We can say that in some cases it is effective.

To sum up the recommendations of this chapter for delaying the skin's aging process:

- Minimize sun exposure.
- Use a sunscreen daily, especially if your skin is Type 1 or 2.
- Wear protective clothing such as hats and blouses with long sleeves. The single most important factor is the tightness of the weave, not the color or thickness of the fabric.
- Plan outdoor activities before 10 A.M. and after 2 P.M. when possible.
- Avoid direct contact with harsh chemicals.
- If it itches, don't scratch.
- Use unscented cosmetics whenever possible.
- Relax!

The rest of the book deals with other ways of delaying the aging process, divided into three categories. First, we discuss home treatment involving soaps, creams, and moisturizers. Then, we examine typical beauty salon programs. Finally, we discuss some of the new procedures available from your dermatologist without surgery to delay and disguise the aging and wrinkling process.

QUESTIONS AND ANSWERS

Q. I've been using sunscreens for many years (my doctor suggested it). But last time out, in just a few minutes, I got a terrible sunburn. What happened?

A. Occasionally people can become sensitive to one of the ingredients in a sunscreen and actually get a photoallergic reaction. It has happened with PABA sunscreens and with others. The only sure way to pin down the cause is to go through the list of ingredients in the product you have been using and have your physician do photo-patch tests. Keep in mind, too, that the ingredients in these sunscreens change all the time. Since they are considered drugs, the law requires that their ingredients be listed on the label.

If we suspect PABA as the culprit, we can go to non-PABA sunscreens like Uval or Maxafil. There's a new non-PABA sunscreen being tested at Harvard Medical School that is also very good about staying on through sweating or swimming. Clinical tests show that, once applied, it does not wash off or sweat off, except with soap and water. It will be available as a lotion, cream, or clear liquid. Of course, other products now make the same claims. Most of the SPF numbers have been calculated with machine-simulated sun and do not take into account such factors as wind, which causes evaporation, and running around, which causes perspiration. This new product is being tested in real live sunlight, and will have a much higher SPF even with this more difficult test. Hitherto unpublished material made available to us leads us to believe that, if the claims are true, we will soon have a much better sunscreen. It will be marketed as Tiscreen.

Q. I want to use a sunscreen but I'm not sure how or when or what type to use. You walk into the market or the drugstore and you see hundreds of them on the shelf. How do you know which one to pick?

A. Good question, and not an easy one to answer. First, you must consider your skin type, which has some bearing on whether you go with a liquid, cream, or gel. Given four sunscreens of equal efficacy, your skin type will help you choose. For instance, if you have oily skin, you would want a sunscreen in an alcohol base, which is drying. You need this especially if you have acne or tend to break out. On the other hand, if you have dry skin that is already sun damaged, you would want a sunscreen in a moisturizer or cream base. That gives you the advantage of the sunscreen plus the advantage of the moisturizer.

Second, you must consider how much protection you want. If you want to get a tan but you still want protection, then you can go with a partial sunscreen instead of a total sunscreen. If you are very fair, you would use an 8 or 10 to allow certain rays to get through, but tan at a slower rate. If you are dark, you can use a lower number. Once you get your tan, go to a higher number to maintain your tan.

Third, you must consider how much activity you will be involved in while using the sunscreen. If you swim or play tennis, you need a sunscreen with substantivity—the ability to avoid washing off. We're not sure there is such a thing at this time, so it's best to reapply the sunscreen often.

A word about the SPF numbers. All the sunscreens now come with these Sun Protection Factor numbers. At this time, the highest possible is supposed to be a 15, even if they have scored higher in tests. Now we all know that some products advertise higher numbers. If it advertises itself as a 19, it might be and it might not be. But what it all comes down to is that, for the most protection, you choose the highest number.

Some sunscreens now carry a seal of approval from the Skin Cancer Foundation of New York, certifying that the product "meets the criteria and standards established by the Skin Cancer Foundation as an effective aid in prevention of sun-induced skin cancer when applied in the prescribed manner." The Skin Cancer Foundation is new but has been active, especially in education to reduce the incidence, morbidity, and mortality of skin cancer throughout the world. They have also established a photobiology committee to standardize procedures for testing sunscreens and to monitor standards in the products they test. Those products that meet the foundation's criteria receive the seal of approval.

Q. Which cosmetics contain sunscreens?

A. There are more every day, at various SPF levels, as the industry comes to realize that sunscreens are the best way to delay the aging process. A by-no-means-complete sampling would include Helena Rubinstein, Texas Pharmaceuticals, Lanvin, Charles of the Ritz, Revson, Revlon, Aida Grey, Tova-9, and Clinique. Given two equal cosmetics, we recommend the one that has the sunscreen.

Q. What about that stuff that's supposed to give you a tan in or out of the sun?

A. You're talking about dihydroxyacetone which, applied to the skin, actually produces a change in color—a shade of brown, but not really the color of tanning. Like the quick tan pills (or the beta-carotene available in health food stores) they cause increased skin color but it's not a natural color and doesn't fool anybody. Nor is it any protection against the sun, since it doesn't involve pigmentation.

Q. Are there pills to make tanning easier?

A. Yes, there are. Presently there are two products available, methoxypsoralen and tripsoralen. (Psoralen was first discovered in Egypt.) If these pills are taken two hours before you go into the sun, they do increase the skin's response to the sun. But they are available only by prescription and are tricky to use. If you get too much sun it can result in *extreme* sunburn with blistering. There's also some question about the long-term safety of these pills. They may be implicated in the development of cataracts. If you use them regularly and get large doses of sun, you get more ultraviolet light damage. Originally they were linked to liver damage, but the latest data suggest that may not be true. When these pills are used to treat certain diseases, they are monitored closely, and that's fine. But we cannot recommend them for every-day tanning. The possible side effects far outweigh any benefits.

Q. How does stress and strain affect aging of the skin?

A. Under stress and strain, people tend to pick up habits like puckering the lips or frowning. The stress of these repeated muscle movements on the underlying collagen will, in time, account for the formation of wrinkles. Most people do not have perfectly symmetrical smiles. The side that grins more usually has more wrinkles.

Q. When should I start worrying about my skin?

A. Yesterday. Long-range skin care should begin in youth and continue throughout life. You should cleanse the surface of the skin daily, use emollients and moisturizers as needed, use sunscreens regularly, and avoid harsh chemicals and perfumed cosmetics. When the time comes, you may want to consider some of the medical procedures discussed later in this book.

In addition, we can list some developments which might signal the time to seek help:

- Any blemish, rash, or change that lingers. (A skin disease that could scar, thicken, or change the face poses an obvious beauty hazard.)
- Any wrinkling around the eyes or mouth, any drying or wrinkling of the skin.
- Bags or puffiness around the eyes.

- Blotchy pigmentation, particularly on the upper lip, cheeks, or forehead.
- Appearance of excessive sun spots or freckles.
- Deepening of the crease between the side of the nose and the mouth.
- Changes in hair, including graying, thinning, and brittleness.
- Redness of the "flush" area (both cheeks and bridge of nose) of the face.
- Double chin or sagging of neck, upper arms, or breast.
- Worry lines reflecting emotional stress.

Q. I have really dry skin. If I eat oily foods or cod liver oil will my skin become oilier?

A. The skin's oiliness is a direct result of the output of the sebaceous glands, which are activated hormonally. Scientific studies suggest that, no matter what you eat, your oil gland output does not change. There's no magic process that can break oil down, race it into your bloodstream, and get it into your oil glands.

Q. What about alcohol and the skin? Does over-indulgence or abuse have an effect?

A. Assuming you and your companions are still seeing straight, you will notice a blotchy redness and a condition known as *rosacea,* which tends to make people look older than they really are. The W.C. Fields look—bulbous nose, red face—is characteristic of the condition which, we should mention before we unjustly accuse anyone, also occurs in people who do not drink. Rosacea-type redness can appear in a butterfly pattern across the cheekbones and over the bridge of the nose when blood vessels have lost their ability to contract. Sun damage can pave the way for this condition. Anything that causes the blood vessels to dilate, such as alcoholic beverages, but also including hot beverages,

spicy foods, and sauna environments, stimulates the redness. It can be treated by coagulating the blood vessels (see
our last chapter) and by avoiding those foods and conditions that bring it on.

*Q. I've had beautiful nails all my life, but all of a sudden they've
become brittle. What happened?*

A. There's not much we can do about life-long brittleness,
but the brittleness that females often get between the age of
thirty-five and fifty usually goes away by itself in a year or
two. If the dermatologist gets the patient at the end of the
two years, he can take credit for the cure. If he gets the
patient at the beginning, somebody else will. It's a natural
phenomenon that nobody seems to understand, but it does
take care of itself.

We can give a few additional hints for general nail
care, though. The most common mistake most people make
is neglect. We recommend a weekly manicure and daily
moisturizing to keep hands, nails, and cuticles conditioned.
We also recommend a nondrying polish remover, since dryness is the chief cause of splits and hangnails. Sometimes
nail varnishes cause damage and changes in color to the
surface of the nail, visible when the polish is removed. You
can scrape the color off yourself. Free formaldehyde is
banned in the United States and we know that it does cause
some nail problems. But it can still be found in some foreign products, and those products should be avoided.

GUIDELINES FOR THE USE OF SUNSCREENS

1.—For maximum resistance to water and perspiration, apply one to two hours before going out in the sun.

2.—Don't forget that you can get burned, even on a cloudy day.

3.—If you are bald, don't forget to use a sunscreen on the head or wear a hat.

4.—Reapply sunscreen every four to five hours and after swimming.

5.—You need more protection at high elevations and in areas where the sand, water, or snow reflects sunlight.

6.—When buying cosmetics, keep in mind those which contain sunscreens.

RECOMMENDATIONS BY SKIN TYPE

For people with Type 1 and 2 skin, we recommend daily use of sunscreens, applied frequently.

For people with Type 3 skin, we recommend sunscreens whenever they expect to be out in the sun longer than a half hour.

For people with Type 4 or 5 skin, we recommend sunscreens only when they plan to spend unusually long periods of time in the sun.

People with Type 6 skin do not need sunscreens.

BELOW ARE THE MOST COMMON SUNSCREEN AGENTS AND THE LIGHT SPECTRUM THEY MOST EFFICIENTLY BLOCK	
PABA and PABA esters	UVB
Cinnamates	UVB
Salicylates	UVB
Anthranilates	UVA, UVB
Benzophenones	UVA, UVB
Opaque products:	UVA, UVB
Titanium dioxide	
Talc	
Zinc oxide	

SOME SUN SCREENS AND THEIR ACTIVE INGREDIENTS

PRODUCT	ACTIVE INGREDIENT	ABSORBS:
Total Eclipse®	PABA ester, oxybenzone	UVB, UVA
Eclipse®	PABA ester, glyceryl PABA	UVB
Pre-Sun 15®	PABA, PABA ester, oxybenzone	UVB, UVA
Pre-Sun 8®	PABA	UVB
Supershade 15®	PABA ester, oxybenzone	UVB, UVA
Piz Buin Exclusive®	Cinnamate, benzophenne	UVB, UVA
Pabanol®	PABA	UVB

PRODUCT	ACTIVE INGREDIENT	ABSORBS:
A-Fil®	menthyl anthranilate, titanium dioxide	UVA, UVB
Sundare®	cinotate	UVB
Sea and Ski 6®	PABA ester	UVB
Sundown Ultra Protection (15)®	PABA ester, oxybenzone	UVA, UVB
Coppertone®	homomenthyl, salicylate	UVB
R V Paque®	red veternarun petrolatum, cinotate, zinc oxide	UVB, UVA
Solbar Plus 15®	PABA ester, oxybenzone	UVB, UVA
Uval®	oxybenzone, p-methoy-cinnamate	UVB, UVA
LIP SUNSCREENS		
Sunstick®	digalloyl trioleates	UVB
Uval Sun'n'Wind Stick®	sulisobenzone	UVB, UVA
RV PABA® Stick	PABA, RVP	UVA, UVB
Chapstick® Sunblock 15	PABA ester, oxybenzone	UVB, UVA
Pre-Sun® Sunscreen Lip protection	PABA ester	UVB
Eclipse® Sunscreen Lip and face protectant	PABA ester	UVB

THREE

Home Skin Care Program: Proper Use of Soaps, Moisturizers, and Cosmetics to Delay Aging

While there are many approaches to keeping your skin looking young, the best place to start is with a well-planned and faithfully executed home skin-care program. Such a program should begin early in life and continue on a regular basis, changing as you get older to tailor itself to your changing needs.

Any skin-care program is a response to potential damage the skin may suffer during a lifetime. In designing a program, we must consider these important factors in aging the skin:

- Overexposure to the sun
- The normal aging process
- Long-term use of irritating or harsh soaps or detergents
- Certain medicated or perfumed creams
- Long-term unprotected exposure to wind and heat
- Overuse and abuse of alcohol
- Certain medications and hormones

• Prolonged tension or emotional disturbances
• Skin growths such as multiple warts, tags, and moles
• Certain diseases, either general or of the skin

Most of us think of aging skin without considering how much is due to the natural aging process and how much is due to these other, sometimes controllable factors. In our youth-oriented society, we often have distorted expectations about how the skin should change as it ages. Before we look at ways to delay the aging process, perhaps it would be helpful to look at what we can realistically expect from the skin as it ages. The best such description we know was written by Herbert J. Spoor of the Cornell University College of Medicine. We summarize it here:

At 20 years, the skin on the face is still free of wrinkles.
At 25, the first wrinkles appear on the forehead and under the eyes. Laugh lines first become apparent.
At 30, crow's feet appear at the corners of the eyes and hair on the upper lip or chin, if previously fuzzy, may grow more obvious.
At 40, permanent wrinkles begin to appear in the area from the ears to the neck.
At 45, the eyes become more sunken and a double chin may appear. The lips become thinner and the eyebrows bushier.
At 50, wrinkles appear around the nose, earlobes, and chin. The skin is noticeably drier.
At 55, folds form at the nape of the neck and, mostly on areas exposed to sunlight, what we call senile hyperpigmentation or discoloration begins.
At 60, wrinkles around the mouth deepen and the cheeks begin to sag. The teeth appear to have grown longer, but in fact the gums have receded.
At 65, hair growth begins or increases in the ear canal, nostrils, neck, and chin.

At 70, wrinkles begin to overlap, forming a criss-crossing net of creases. The hair on the scalp gets thinner. Pigmentation is now quite evident.

We'll spare you the description of the skin between 75 and 80, but you get the picture. The changes described by Dr. Spoor are average. They may come sooner or they may come later. Genetic influences play an important role, but care of the skin is equally important. If we carefully examine the items on the first list, the factors in aging the skin, we may be able to delay the effects described in the second list, above.

The most important item on the first list, as we have mentioned before, is overexposure to the sun's rays. It cannot be overemphasized that sun damage starts from a child's first exposure to the sun, that it is cumulative, and that it is irreversible. At what age sun damage begins to be noticeable on the skin depends on three factors—(1) the amount of exposure to the sun; (2) the intensity of the exposure (the sun, for example, is more intense at the equator than at the North Pole); and (3) your skin type, which is determined by your genes. Once you have accumulated "enough" sun damage, the solar keratoses and sun spots you develop will continue to develop, even if you never expose yourself to the sun again, albeit at a slower rate. But don't let that mislead you. You may not avoid the damage that has already been done if you stay out of the sun. But you can avoid causing more damage and, even at that late date, you can take precautions. Protecting your skin against the sun is a crucial part of skin care at any age.

Other factors merit a brief mention. Alcohol may not seem especially relevant to skin care until we consider how easy it is to recognize the alcoholic face—and how unflattering it is. Hyperpigmentation is familiar to women who have given birth, but others may not be aware that these changes on the face are not only associated with pregnancy. They can also be the result of estrogen, either taken alone or in the Pill. We are all familiar, of course, with the lines around the eyes, on the forehead, and around the mouth that can be caused by tension.

In this chapter, we will discuss soaps and moisturizers. While soaps and other cleansing agents seldom have anything to do with permanent cosmetic changes, it is important to use them properly. Over the years, continual use of specific soaps and detergents can dry out the skin, aggravate already dry skin, and be responsible for a dry skin condition, which lasts longer than it should. Some people may find one of the numerous "dry skin" soaps on the market is the answer to the problem, while others may find that they have to give up soap entirely in favor of cleansing creams, soap substitutes, or nothing but plain water. Moisturizers play a definite role in any home skin-care program and, since they are usually not well understood by the layman, will receive special attention.

SOAP

Whoever first said that cleanlinesss is next to godliness did not have dry skin. Dry skin does not cause wrinkles, but there is no question that it makes them more noticeable. Some soaps can be a cause of dry skin. Improper use of soap—or using the improper soap—can significantly contribute to the problems of aging skin.

The average American goes through more than twenty-eight pounds of soaps and detergents each year. This is far more cleanliness than anyone except a major deity requires. A high percentage of the patients we see are concerned about the right way to clean their faces. Upon examination we often find that their concern was justified. Many of them are using either the wrong methods or the wrong products.

Americans bathe too often—especially those who live in a cold climate, have prematurely sun-damaged skin, or are advanced in years. While the use of soap goes back to the ancient Phoenicians, it was not until the eighteenth century that it became popular for use on the human body. Some of us may remember our mothers or grandmothers making soap at home, heating natural fats (with an excess of sodium hydroxide) in an open kettle, adding salt when the reaction was complete, and waiting for the soap to congeal. The result was lye soap, one of the harshest types of soap one could use.

Although modern manufacturing methods reduce the alkalinity to neutral or slightly acidic, remove impurities, and thus considerably lower the soap's tendency to irritate, the process is still essentially the same. All soaps are potential skin irritants. They will dry out the skin because of the way they work.

Soap, a compound formed by the action of fats and alkalis, is by nature alkaline in pH. It has the ability to hook onto dirt, debris, and oil, make them water soluble, and send them down the drain. In scientific terms, soap is an alkali-metal salt of long-chain fatty acids. One end of the chain is positively charged and will mix with water; the other end is nonpolar and, thus, able to surround the dirt, debris, and oil. It is here that we encounter our first problem with soap. It cannot tell the difference between the oils we would like to wash down the drain and the natural oils of the skin that we would like to keep right where they are. Hence, when we use soap to wash away the grime, we also wash away some of the essential oils that are needed as a protective sealing layer for the skin. Without that protection, the skin when exposed to evaporation and towel drying, will lose its moisture and will dry out.

When we talk about dry skin, we refer specifically to the water content of the stratum corneum, the outermost layer of the skin. As the result of physical or chemical stimuli, the stratum corneum can thicken. As it thickens, it becomes less flexible. Dehydration adds to the loss of flexibility. Frequent use of soap and hot water provides both physical and chemical stimuli.

How do we prevent dryness and thickening of the skin? One way is to remove these harsh stimuli. In this section we will recommend a series of procedures which, if followed regularly, will decrease or eliminate this problem.

The use of mild, nonirritating cleansing products is sometimes easier said than done. The manufacturers of bar soap are not required by law to list their ingredients on the label. Thus, a bar soap, unless otherwise labeled, may be a true soap, a detergent (that is, made of synthetic or man-made chemicals), or a combination of the two. Detergents clean basically the same way soaps do but, since they are more efficient at removing surface oil, they are also a little more drying. Detergents are also less alkaline than soaps and are not affected by hard water. Mild or neutral soaps and detergents are easier on dry, aging, and sun-damaged skin. "Super-fatted" soaps may be a little milder than regular soaps, but are also less efficient.

How do we choose the right soap then from the hundreds of brands available? It's largely a matter of trial and error, but we can narrow it down considerably by discussing the different types of skin texture. (These skin texture types are not the same as the skin types described in the chapter, "Delaying the Aging Process" for use with sunscreens.)

SKIN TEXTURE TYPES

Group 1. Light complexion, little natural oil, thin skin, occasional freckles, light-sensitive, sunburns easily, sometimes red hair and ruddy complexion.

Group 2. "Normal" skin, i.e. moderate thickness, oil glands sufficient to keep skin lubricated and flexible, tolerates sun in average doses, tans easily.

Group 3. Heavy, thick skin, usually brunette with generally brown skin, many oil glands, rarely sunburns.

People in Group 3 need to wash their faces thoroughly with a soap or detergent, sometimes two or three times daily.

People in Group 2 may need to wash their faces once or twice a day and use cleansing cream and moisturizers. They can probably use a regular soap without danger of irritation.

People in Group 1 must be very careful of their skin, using cleansing creams and moisturizers and avoiding the sun. They may experiment with any of the neutral or slightly acidic soaps or detergents. All soaps, cold creams, and moisturizers should be unscented and unmedicated—except for the addition of a sunscreen to moisturizers.

Some people have such sensitive skin that they can tolerate only water or a waterless cleanser, such as Cetaphil® lotion, for cleansing. Since these people have almost no natural oil, liberal use of moisturizers is imperative.

We recommend any of the following soaps for people in Group 1 or people who have had problems finding a nonirritating soap: Dove®, Emulave® or Aveenobar® (oatmeal), Lowila®, Oilatum®, Purpose®, and Neutrogena®. Try several—you are the best judge of which you prefer. We recommend neutral or mildly acidic soaps, since the skin has an acid pH and most soaps are alkaline. We also recommend soap substitutes, made with oatmeal or starch. Even these, however, can be irritating to some people, especially those in Group 1. What makes some soaps more irritating than others is still not completely clear. Additives like cholesterol, fatty acid, and lanolin do not, incidentally, seem to help much, because the soap's cleansing action also washes away these additives.

If you use a cleansing cream, we also recommend that it be neutral or mildly acid. Perfumed cleansing creams are unnecessary and undesirable, as are creams with cooling chemicals. There is little difference between a cleansing cream and a cold cream. The function of both is similar to soap—to cleanse the skin. The ingredients of cleansing and cold creams liquefy the fatty secretions on the skin and pick up particles of dirt and debris, which can then be wiped off with soft tissues or a soft towel. Creams are also highly efficient for removing oily makeup. Chemically, cleansing creams are emulsions, usually water in oil base (that is, more oil than water).

By now, the reason we have devoted so much space to soap in a book about the management of aging skin should be apparent. Dryness and wrinkling are part of the aging process. Proper care of the facial skin can increase moisturization, thus combatting dryness and making wrinkles less noticeable. Conversely, improper care of the face can make it look years older than it has to. The proper use of soap, moisturizers, and even cosmetics is essential to maintaining a youthful appearance.

To sum up our recommendations for the use of soap:

• Use the chart above to determine which group your skin texture belongs to. Group 1 should use very mild soaps or cleansing creams, use moisturizers liberally, completely avoid unprotected exposure to the sun. Group 2 should use mild soaps moderately (once or twice a day), cleansing creams if desired, and moisturizers as needed. Moderate sun exposure is permissible if a sun block is used. Group 3 should use soap two or three times a day as needed to remove oil. Sun exposure is permissible.

- Treat older, drier skin as Group 1.
- Soaps and cleansing agents should be neutral or slightly acidic.
- Cleansing creams are recommended for removing oily makeup.

MOISTURIZERS

The most important thing to understand about moisturizers is that they do not moisturize. Only water can moisturize skin enough to enhance its elasticity. Moisturizers work by helping the skin retain water. The more water in the skin, the more it stretches and puffs up, making small wrinkles and crow's feet less visible.

Oil alone does not make the skin pliable. The classic demonstration of this was an experiment by Dr. Irving Blank, who took two pieces of dry, hard human callus and soaked one piece in water and the other in oil. The results were dramatic. The oil did not moisturize. The water did.

Theoretically, there are two ways to help the skin retain water. One is to use some kind of substance that would attract and hold water. It is questionable whether this substance exists. The other is to apply something to seal the skin and act as a physical barrier to prevent evaporation of water from the skin. The natural oils of your face are helpful for this task if they are not removed by washing with soap. After toweling and evaporation, your face is actually drier than before you washed it.

Petrolatum is very effective at reducing water loss, but most people do not like to be that greasy, except possibly at night. Oil-in-water emulsions (lotions and vanishing cream) are the most popular moisturizers. Water-in-oil emulsions as well as petrolatum may bring about an acneform eruption in some people that is known appropriately as acne cosmetica. There is one simple and obvious cure for acne cosmetica, and that is to switch cosmetics. If you are prone to breaking out, look for the water-based preparation instead of the oil-based. (Most companies make both versions.) A quick test of your present moisturizers or cosmetics will tell you whether they are water-based or oil-based. Spread a little on the palm of your hand. If, as the water evaporates, you feel a cooling sensation, the emulsion is water based, that is, a substance with more water than oil. If your hand feels warm, the emulsion is oil based. The preparation with more oil absorbs more warmth from your body. For people who tend to break out when they use moisturizers, we recommend using one with little or no lanolin, mineral oil, isopropyl myristate, cocoa butter, or sodium lauryl sulfate. Such a preparation may not be easy to find. We suggest Shepard's lotion or cream (unscented).

While, as we mentioned, some believe a substance that would increase the skin's ability to absorb water does not exist, some moisturizers do claim to contain such a substance, which is called a humectant. Of the natural humectants, lactic acid, sodium pyrrolidone carboxylic acid, and urea seem to be the most effective, though there is some reason to suspect long-term use of urea may damage the stratum corneum. Other substances often listed as humectants include glycerin, propylene glycol, and butylene glycol. These natural humectants reach the skin via the sweat glands; they include lactic acid, urea, sodium chloride (salt), and sodium pyrrolidone carboxylic acid.

In dry climates, the skin loses moisture through the air. A relative humidity above 30 to 40 percent is enough to keep the skin moist, but anything below that will cause the kind of dryness that is often called "winter itch." This can be combatted by using less soap, bathing less often, and bathing for a shorter time. Moisturizers will also help, as will the use of humidifiers to restore moisture to the air. Increasing the moisture will help the itching so common in older and sun-damaged skin and, of course, make small wrinkles less noticeable.

When it comes to choosing moisturizers and cosmetics, please keep in mind that a product is not superior just because it is expensive. Manufacturers are now required by the Food and Drug Administration to list their ingredients on the label in order of decreasing percentage. (Soap is exempt from the ruling.) It is quite possible to find that two products, which differ greatly in cost, contain exactly the same ingredients. One of our favorite moisturizers can be easily and inexpensively mixed at home—equal parts of petrolatum and aquaphor, both available without a prescription. For those not interested in playing chemist, we can recommend U-Lactin™, Aquacare®/HP, Lacticare® lotion, or Keri® lotion, to mention a few.

There are a number of additives you probably do not need. They are exotic and decorative—and they drive the price up. Despite cosmetic companies' testimonials for royal bee jelly, aloe vera, ginseng, oil of turtle, RNA, DNA, polypeptides, and jojoba, *ad nauseum,* there are as yet no scientific studies to suggest that any of these additives are effective. Protein or collagen may add to the sealing power of a moisturizer, but it is important to note that they do not penetrate the skin deeply enough to have any impact on your body's own protein or collagen. Used on the surface, collagen has no long-term effect on wrinkles. Collagen is only effective for wrinkles when implanted by injection, which we discuss in Chapter Ten.

Bath oils also aid in moisturizing. The many brands available fall essentially into two types. One contains emulsifiers that disperse in the water, theoretically adding a sealing layer to your moistened skin. The other forms a film on the surface of the water. As you get out of the bath, the film will stick to the surface of your moistened skin. For baths, follow the directions on the bottle. For showers, apply them while the skin is still wet, then towel dry. Bath oils can be used in combination with moisturizers, which is especially recommended in dry, cold climates and in winter.

The best way to use a moisturizer is to apply it to moist skin. Wash or bathe; then apply the moisturizer before the skin has a chance to dry out.

To sum up the recommendations of this chapter for use of moisturizers:

- Moisturizers have no long-term effect on the skin.
- Moisturizers do have a definite short-term effect on the skin. They reduce dryness and, by helping the skin retain water, make small wrinkles less noticeable.
- Additives add to the price, not to the quality of most moisturizers. One exception is a sunscreen added to a moisturizer, which will have a long-term effect.
- Moisturizers should be applied when the skin is moist. The object is to trap water in the skin.
- If you have a tendency to break out, you must choose your moisturizer with care, as described in this chapter.

COSMETICS

There is no shortage of books on how cosmetics can hide wrinkles. For a long time that was the only method available. There is no point in our rehashing that here. But, since we are offering an alternative to both cosmetics and plastic surgery, it may be helpful to suggest how cosmetics can be used to hide the immediate effects of surgery and the less drastic procedures we describe in Chapters Six, Seven, Eight, and Nine. We might call this "corrective cosmetics."

Most users of cosmetics do not understand the art of concealing unwanted features. In most cases, they have never needed to. They have used cosmetics to make aged skin look better, an attempt to make wrinkles less noticeable, to cover "sun spots" or dark circles under the eyes, or to hide flabbiness by using shading for contour. Cosmetic surgery and cosmetic office procedures may present a new challenge—to conceal discoloration or scar tissue immediately after the procedure and, if necessary, over the long run.

Suppose a procedure has left, temporarily, a red scar or a large bruise. A spot cover or concealing preparation is usually recommended. Thick and pastelike, it is applied with the fingers like finger paint. Don't pull or stretch the skin when applying these, and be particularly careful under the eyes. As your body temperature warms the preparation, use the pads of the fingertips to blend it in naturally. After it dries, you may apply more as needed. This technique works especially well for large circles under the eyes. First, cleanse the skin. Then apply the concealor, which should be slightly lighter than your skin color. When it dries, apply your foundation or face makeup over the lighter area and blend it in, being careful not to leave lines of demarcation between the different shades.

A hematoma (a raised area caused by blood under the skin) can be concealed the same way. Whether it is the result of a cosmetic procedure or bumping into a door, the discolored swelling is not something you will want to display to the world. Start, again, with light fingertip application. The pain will remind you to be gentle. Let it dry and set, then apply a second coat until the camouflage is complete. Blend, using more than one shade if necessary. If the hematoma is on a hand, it may present more of an artistic challenge since there are more hills and valleys of bone and contour that produce shadows. The need to also camouflage sun spots may complicate the process, but a color blender into the areas of shadows combined with concealors can work wonders.

Scars come in all sizes, shapes, colors, and—unfortunately—places. One thing they all have in common is that they are different from normal skin. They contain no hair, hair follicles, or pores. They may have no color or too much color (hypopigmentation as opposed to hyperpigmentation), but they can be made less noticeable. You may find that your usual makeup will not adhere to a scar. You may need to turn to a greaseless preparation. If the scar is depressed, several applications may be required in order to fill it in. Using a lighter-than-skin-tone color on indented areas also has the effect of making them look full. Used in stick form, a small amount can be applied and effectively blended so that no line of demarcation is evident.

Successful blending is absolutely essential to the final outcome. With a little practice, it is easy. The lines of demarcation should be practically invisible. What lines do appear should be used to good effect. Lines running downward tend to accentuate frowns and age. Upward lines accentuate smiles, youth, and happiness. (Were that all of life were this simple!) Highlighter, a preparation lighter than your own skin color, is useful for postoperative swelling. A well-blended line of highlighter down the center of a swollen nose creates an effective illusion, making the defect less noticeable.

Smile lines, frown lines, and grooves around the mouth or on the forehead will bring out the artist in you. Use a fine brush to draw a thin line down the center of the groove. Use the fingertips to blend, assuring that there is highlighter only in the groove, not on the flat surface of the skin. Only the indented area should be lighter in color. For contouring, it's just the opposite. Use a color darker than your skin tone to create the illusion of shadows. Shadows in an area of swelling or asymmetry can balance the contours of the face by creating the illusion that the swollen area recedes. Contouring under the jaw can camouflauge a lax neck or jowls. Contouring is most effective when used in conjunction with highlighting.

Face makeup or foundation, which comes in many forms and colors, can be used to minimize or hide unwanted blemishes and pigmentary changes. Normally, your makeup is supposed to match your skin color. But if your skin is sallow or yellowish, try a mauve or pink-toned base. If your skin is red or ruddy (often a result of sun damage or over-indulgence in alcohol), try a light green tinted moisturizer or base followed by beige makeup. For local areas of solar keratoses—those rough, reddish lesions most commonly found on the face—this can also be effective, toning down the redness considerably.

The cosmetics industry thrives by playing on our preoccupation with youthfulness and attractiveness, using the time-honored approach of the carrot and the stick. If we are still youthful, they tempt us by promising we can be more attractive. If we are not youthful, they promise us at least a youthful appearance. This scheme works splendidly as long as we accept their premises. We would suggest, however, that not everyone likes or needs carrots.

To summarize:

- Use of opaque and/or translucent color on the skin can effectively create desired shadows and highlights to conceal unwanted defects.
- We mentioned product types available at most cosmetic counters, but it is not necessary to use any particular brand.
- Horizontal lines make the face look wider.
- Vertical or diagonal lines make the face look thinner.

QUESTIONS AND ANSWERS

Q. What is the difference between a cold cream and a cleansing cream?

A. Cleansing creams are just a variation of the original cold cream ingredients. Both serve the same purpose. And

what makes a cold cream cold? Usually a chemical like menthol.

Q. Do we bathe too often?

A. We think so. As we get older, the skin does not function
as well. It gets thinner; it contains less water, and the oil
glands secrete less actively. Add to that the dehydration
and defatting of the skin that comes with bathing, and you
are asking for trouble. As we get older dry skin is a common cause of itching and, while it may not cause wrinkles,
it certainly accentuates them.

*Q. What is the difference between detergents and soaps, especially
regarding their effect on the skin?*

A. Although the words soap and detergent are often used
interchangeably, there are some differences. Soaps are made
from natural fats and oils. Detergents are made from synthetic, or man-made, chemicals. Both remove water-soluble
oils, but detergents are usually more efficient as cleansers
and less affected by hard water. Unfortunately, they also
have a higher alkali content and thus are more likely to dry
and irritate the skin.

Q. Are all detergents more irritating than soap?

A. If you decrease the irritancy of a detergent with additives like synthetic fillers, you also decrease its efficiency.
By special chemical processes detergents can be made neutral or mildly acidic, and hence, less irritating.

Q. Why does my soap leave a film on my skin?

A. Soaps made from natural substances do tend to leave a
precipitate when they encounter the calcium, magnesium,
or ferric ions found in hard water. If you live in a hard
water area, you may be better off (film-wise, at least) with a
detergent.

Q. Which antibacterial soap do you recommend and is it true that they are very drying?

A. People with normal skin can usually tolerate any soap on the market. But if soaps do cause irritation you may be interested in a recent study that rated Dove®, Aveenobar®, Purpose®, Dial®, and Alpha Keri® the least irritating of eighteen well-known soaps tested. Of these, only Dial® contains an antibacterial agent.

Q. The soap ads say cholesterol, fatty acids, and lanolin help make a soap more moisturizing. Is that true?

A. Probably not. Whatever emollients are added to the soap are subject to the same cleaning action as dirt. They usually wash off before they can do the job.

Q. When is the best time to moisturize your body?

A. Directly after bathing, because that's when your skin has the most moisture in it, in the form of water. If you then apply a moisturizer, it leaves a semi-permeable cover on the skin that traps the moisture in and keeps the skin pliable for a longer period of time. But any time your skin feels dry or uncomfortable you can use a moisturizer.

Q. How come some parts of my face feel oily and other parts feel dry? Can a person have oily and dry skin at the same time?

A. There is a higher concentration of oil glands in the central part of the face—between the eyebrows, around the nose, down the chin, and into the "V" of the neck—than elsewhere, and these areas are usually oiler.

Q. What is lanolin and what does it do?

A. Lanolin is a liquid or fat that is secreted by the sebaceous glands of sheep. Extracted from the hair of sheep, refined and purified, it is used in many cosmetics, creams, lotions, and medical preparations as a lubricant. Not only is it a very good lubricant, it also serves as a moisturizer. Some people are allergic to lanolin, which makes them break out.

Q. What do you think of hormone or estrogen creams?

A. Since estrogens are readily absorbed through the skin, these creams can only contain a very small amount of any active ingredient if they are to be safe. In fact, they contain so little estrogen that the most it can do is cause a slight swelling of the skin–but that may be due more to the cream itself than the additive. The swelling does make wrinkles less noticeable (temporarily).

Q. Which moisturizers do you recommend for people who break out?

A. We suggest a water-based as opposed to an oil-based moisturizer. Some companies make both such as Clinique, Charles of the Ritz, Coty, Dermik, Elizabeth Arden, Ponds, Revlon, and Yardley, to name a few.

Q. What is the difference between a moisturizer and a wrinkle cream?

A. Wrinkle cream is no longer a legally acceptable term. The Federal Trade Commission has issued many cease and desist orders to companies claiming their creams can remove wrinkles. And that's good; the term should be a thing of the past. To think a cream exists that would not only stop the aging process but reverse it is pure folly. The onset of wrinkles may be delayed. Their appearance may be temporarily improved with emollients or moisturizers. But, to date, there is no fountain of youth that comes in a jar.

Q. What causes rough skin and what can be done about it?

A. Skin is a living organ that is constantly renewing itself. New cells grow up from the lower levels and slough off at the top. In the best of all worlds, they would all slough off at the same time and we would all have lovely, smooth skin. Unfortunately, that doesn't happen. They come off in different areas at different rates and sometimes only partially, clinging to the surface and forming flakes. These flakes of partially detached cells protrude above the surface of the skin and make it rough to the touch. Soaps, detergents, water, and cleansers irritate the upper layer of the skin, resulting in frequent hydration and swelling. This irritation loosens and displaces the stratum corneum. There are two ways to treat the problem. Oil containing moisturizers or emollients will take care of the problem if it is not too severe. Otherwise, keratolytic agents can be used to dissolve the rough material. Keratolytics in the form of creams or lotions containing lactic acid, urea, or salycylic acid soften the rough layer and make it easily removable by mechanical means.

Q. Do you consider moisturizers for the face a cosmetic option or a must?

A. Moisturizers should be used only if needed. There was an interesting study of oily skin in which the researchers took one small area, defatted it completely using ether, and then weighed the material they removed. Knowing the weight of the ether and other materials used, they could then figure the weight of the oil they had removed. The next day, they repeated the procedure—and removed the same amount of oil. So it appears that the skin provides a constant output of oil and sheds only the excess. If you have oily skin and do nothing to dehydrate it or dry it out, there is no reason to use a moisturizer. But if you have dry skin, it is important to keep the skin hydrated by the use of moisturizers.

Q. I've seen products advertised that claim to be "biologically active," to "oxygenate" the skin cells, even to accelerate

*the activity of the basal cell layer. Is there any truth to these
claims?*

A. Any product that changes the structure and function of
the skin cannot go by the name cosmetic. The Food and
Drug Administration would classify it as a drug and subject it to manufacturing, advertising, and labeling restrictions. If a product makes such a claim, it should have evidence on file that is open to public inspection—studies that
have been done to verify the claims. In fact, most of these
so-called medicated cosmetics contain such miniscule
amounts of any active ingredient that, even if the ingredient were absorbed, it would be hard to prove it had any
effect on the structure and function of the skin.

Q. What causes bags under the eyes?

A. Bags under the eyes can be due to several causes. Hay
fever, chronic dermatitis, sinusitis, or any local irritant or
allergic reaction can cause the eyelids to swell. The connective tissue under the skin of the lower lids makes it an ideal
place for pooling and slow release of tissue fluids, often referred to as *edema.* Edema is often apparent in the morning, but once you get out of bed and gravity causes the pool
to drain back into the system, it disappears. But most people, when they talk about bags under their eyes, mean the
chronic pouches that tend to occur in older individuals.
These come in two varieties. In the first, the skin stretches
and thins and soon resembles crumpled-up tissue paper.
This is caused by changes in elasticity due to aging and sun
damage. In the second, fibrous tissues beneath the skin
relax, allowing subcutaneous fat to protrude through the
lax bands of connective tissue and take up residence in a
"bag" just under the skin. The best treatment for this is
plastic surgery.

*Q. What causes dark circles under the eyes? Do they indicate
anything wrong physically?*

A. Since the skin under the eyes is thin, it is often possible to see the underlying network of small veins returning blue blood to the heart. These become more prominent when the person is ill, tired, pale, or has lost a great deal of weight. Increase in skin pigment can also cause dark areas under the eyes. Both conditions are in part hereditary.

Q. How can I be having a reaction to the cosmetic I use when I've been using the same one for years?

A. The answer to this is two-fold. First, you are not born allergic to anything. You *become* allergic to something after using it for some time, as the body comes to recognize the item as foreign. Second, cosmetics companies often change the ingredients or the proportion of ingredients in a product without changing its name. All of a sudden, the cosmetic that you've used for years has a new ingredient in it. But if we consider how many women use cosmetics and how many cosmetics are on the market, the incidence of allergic reaction we see is really very low.

Q. I have a feeling of tightness and dry skin on my face. What is causing this?

A. It could be a number of things. Drying due to aging and sun damage. Overuse of soaps and detergents. Overuse of certain cosmetics, especially astringents, clarifying lotions, toners, and fresheners, all of which have high alcohol content, and hence, are drying. Once you figure out which of these is the cause, you can stop using it. Moisturizing cream will also help.

Q. I have itching of the face, yet I don't seem to have broken out.

A. We may well find, if we examine you closely, that you have not broken out. You may be allergic to some perfume that, even in the smallest of doses, triggers your reaction, and the perfume may be in a shampoo or cologne—or even worn by somebody else.

Q. My dermatologist is always recommending that I use water-based makeup, but the few I have tried always seem to be very chalky. Where can I find one I like?

A. Since individual tastes vary, the best we can suggest is that you shop around. Most companies do make both a water- and an oil-based line.

Q. Is there some way to make sure a cosmetic or moisturizer is oil-free?

A. Check the list of ingredients for any animal, vegetable, or mineral oils such as fatty derivatives that have been made hydrophylic through various chemical processes, fatty alcohols, emulsifiers, and hydrophylic gums. See the Glossary on how to read a cosmetics label.

FOUR

Hair

The ancient Hindus spent a great deal of time worrying about how to keep their hair out of the hands of wizards, who could use it to gain power over them. French peasants and Chilean gauchos bury their shorn hair and mark the spot, hoping to take it with them when they are resurrected on Judgement Day. Some cultures think shaving the hair is an act of purification. Others think you can turn a woman's hair into snakes by burying it in horse dung. Our own obsession with shampoos, conditioners, and hair restorers is tame by comparison—but probably of no less concern.

We know what happens as the hair grows old. It gets brittle, thins, turns gray, and, in some cases, falls out. What can we do to prevent that?

HAIR LOSS

First, we are happy to allay some common fears. Most complaints about hair loss that we get in our office are not cases of impending baldness but mere evidence that the hair is replacing itself normally. Hair is a dead structure. No matter how much "life" you manage to put into it, it is made up of one hundred thousand totally dead keratin fibers, and the hair is constantly turning over. A single hair lasts two to six years and is then replaced. Thus, a loss of eighty to one hundred hair a day and twice that much after shampooing or vigorous brushing is completely normal.

True hair loss begins, if it is going to begin, at thirty or thirty-five years of age and continues gradually through the sixties. In men, it may start earlier, as early as the late teens, and result in the typical androgenic male pattern baldness. Younger women are generally protected from androgenic baldness by the presence of estrogen. But as they get older and production of estrogen decreases they may lose 20 to 50 percent of their hair. It is very rare for women to go completely bald.

Any product that claims to grow hair or prevent baldness would be banned if a current Food and Drug Administration proposal is adopted, and any new products would have to prove their safety and effectiveness to the FDA before being allowed on the market. The FDA proposed its ban after an advisory panel reported that none of the products that claimed to grow hair or prevent baldness were effective. (These products usually contain lanolin, olive oil, wheat germ oil, or vitamins.) On the subject of sex hormones taken internally to stimulate growth, the panel said that they could in fact stimulate hair growth—but not necessarily in the right places. The only satisfactory treatment we know of for baldness is a surgical procedure, the hair transplant, which is done not only on men but also on women whose hair is thinning. (The hair transplant for women is still rare.)

From our unbiased viewpoint, it seems that most people exaggerate the extent of their hair loss. We frequently see people who fear they have lost "at least 50 percent" of their hair. Now, as we mentioned, 50 percent is the most a woman can usually expect to lose and when 50 percent of the hair is gone, you can see through the hair to the scalp from the hairline to the crown. Most of these people have lost 5 to 10 percent of their hair at the most. Some of them have lost none.

BRITTLENESS AND BREAKING

Brittleness usually results from over manipulating the hair, be it with chemicals, bleach, dye, overvigorous brushing and combing, combing wet hair, back combing, teasing, ironing, or (how could we leave this out?) too much exposure to the sun. Since hair is a dead structure, it has no means of repairing itself. Abuse leads to breaking and frayed ends and makes the hair more vulnerable to continued damage. Hair that has been dyed or bleached is more susceptible to sun damage than it would be had it stayed its natural color—especially if that natural color was dark. Sun exposure, as does mechanical trauma, accumulates. We know of few shampoos that contain sunscreens and no studies of whether the active chemicals would stick to the hair. But we are surprised that some enterprising cosmetics company has not yet studied the effects of using a PABA rinse for the hair.

GRAYING

Gray hair is one of the most obvious signs of aging. Over the years, the pigment in the hair gradually dilutes, passing slowly through all the tones between natural and white. While no one is certain at this point, the feeling is that a decrease of tyrosinase activity in the melanocytes of the hair bulbs brings on the loss of pigment. Tyrosinase is an enzyme instrumental in the development of pigmented melanin, and melanin is what gives skin and hair its color.

If you look at white hair through an electron microscope, you will see few if any melanin pigment granules.

When your hair starts turning gray is a matter of heredity, unless it is due to hyperthyroidism or cardiovascular disease. White hairs generally appear first at the temples and then slowly spread over the rest of the scalp. Graying of the beard and body hair usually comes later, while pubic and axillary hair may take much longer to turn gray. The age of onset varies by race—thirty to forty in whites and Orientals, thirty-five to fifty-five in blacks. If your hair seems to have turned gray overnight, what probably happened was that you already had both white and black hairs when, perhaps due to a scalp disease, all the black hairs fell out at once leaving only white hairs.

As you probably suspected, there is no antidote for graying hair. In studies done many years ago, some patients who took large doses of PABA internally recovered their normal hair color, but we cannot recommend that treatment at this time. And we've all seen the ads for Grecian Formula®, where little by little gray hair turns back into an allegedly normal color. Grecian Formula® contains a lead acetate in an aqueous solution in small amounts of precipitated sulfur. It is used daily but nothing happens for about a month, when lead sulfide plus oxide appears on the hair shaft, producing color. There are both men's and women's preparations.

GENERAL HAIR CARE

We don't mean to paint too bleak a picture. There are some very worthwhile ways to give hair a younger and

---

Vath, William R. "Are American Women Becoming Bald?" in *Todays Health.* (American Medical Association, January, 1962).

healthier appearance. Most of them were summarized best some years ago in *Today's Health:*

1.–Good general health is most important. Keep fit, get enough sleep, and eat a balanced diet.

2.–Brush moderately, forgetting about the old rule of one hundred strokes daily, unless you have long, thick hair. Some specialists advise a gentle five- to ten-minute massage each day instead of brushing.

3.–Shampoo regularly. This means once a week for most women. Adolescents and women with oily hair should shampoo more frequently.

4.–Don't dry your hair by rubbing briskly with a towel; use a dryer which can be carefully regulated to avoid overheating.

5.–If you have dry hair, shampoo less frequently and avoid the use of bleaches. Use permanent waves less often. Most women get too many permanents, especially after menopause, when the hair becomes drier.

6.–Don't play with your hair or comb it constantly throughout the day. Don't use the ponytail style.

7.–If you find you are losing more than the normal amount of hair, mention it to your hairdresser and tell him to handle your hair gently. Don't let him pull it very tightly to achieve a certain type of set.

8.–Don't be misled by advertising for creams, tonics, medications which offer glowing promises of relief for thinning hair. No amount of advertising will persuade the scalp to grow hair simply because some patent medicine is rubbed into it.

9.–If you become aware of increased hair loss, don't panic. Remember, it is often temporary. If, however, you notice a definite thinning, consult a dermatologist.

The future does offer hope. Some of the best minds (housed beneath some of the baldest scalps?) are testing new products all the time. An antihypertensive drug that seemed to be accompanied by new hair growth in certain areas is now being tested as a local solution for hair loss.

Anti-androgens used topically in the area of hair loss are being tested, but the results so far are not promising. Injection or application of a topical progesterone compound on the scalp is also under investigation.

And there are a couple of new products that actually do live up to their claims of making the hair more manageable and building body. In protein shampoo, the polypeptides obtained from animal collagen soak through the hair shaft and stick to the inside wall of the shaft, adding body and helping to remove split ends. Henna, which has been around for thousands of years as an orange-red hair dye, now comes as a clear additive in shampoo and gives hair body by clinging to the hair shaft.

A number of these preparations are available over the counter and we recommend giving them a try. Some people think they work. Some people don't. You'll know in a hurry whether they work for you.

QUESTIONS AND ANSWERS

Q. If any one hair is only present on the head from two to six years, then how can your hair grow old? That is, why is any hair older than six years?

A. This is partly true, but other factors are at work. The hair may not be older than six years, but the hair bulb is. Its function changes as you grow older and your hormonal patterns change. The hair does not grow as fast. Since melanocyte activity slows, the hair color changes. The oil glands slow down, so less oil gets onto the hair as you brush to give it texture and protect it from the environment.

Q. Does hair style have anything to do with hair loss?

A. Yes, in fact there is even a medical term for hair loss due to mechanical strain. We call it *traction alopecia,* which can be caused by ponytails, braiding, curling, rollers, and bobby pins, all of which constantly pull on the hair shaft. If this goes on long enough, it can actually result in permanent hair loss with scarring of the follicles, usually at the front or back of the scalp or around the ears. The solution is simple: just change the hair style. If you must use rollers, don't pull them too tight.

Q. Will shampooing hurt my hair or slow its growth?

A. Hair, like other structures, varies from person to person. If you have dry hair, over-shampooing will make it drier, and hence, less manageable and lustrous. But it should be remembered that the only "live" part of the hair structure is the part growing in the hair follicle, which is safely nestled about three millimeters below the stratum corneum, a good protective barrier. Shampooing and cleaning do not affect that part of the hair structure, and that is the only part involved in hair growth.

Q. Why am I losing my hair?

A. Usually when we hear this question from women, it turns out they are not losing their hair at all. What happens is that they suddenly notice the hair's natural loss of eighty to a hundred hairs a day. In a study of one hundred and fifty women who thought they were losing their hair, in 45 percent of them no cause was found. In 25 percent, the cause was found to be endocrine in nature, mostly thyroid disease. In less than 5 percent, the hair loss was hereditary and in 25 percent, it was the result of systemic abnormalities. In another study, involving one hundred patients with a diffuse type of hair loss, 20 percent of them were found to be iron deficient without being anemic and, following iron therapy, hair loss stopped. Certain types of hair loss can be treated and reversed.

Q. Does vigorous scalp massage make the hair grow back?

A. Plenty of bald people have tried it. We might note that when we do hair transplants and remove plugs of growing, functioning hair from the side of the scalp to replant on the top, the hair grows just fine. If the reason for the original hair loss in that location was lack of circulation, you would think that the new hair would also die. Not so.

Q. Is it true that henna makes the hair look thicker?

A. Henna has been around for thousands of years as a dye. Unfortunately, it's approximately the color of a carrot, and not too many people find that attractive in hair. The new, colorless henna seems to increase the shine on the hair as well as increase body and the diameter of individual hairs. Unfortunately, they also make the hair stiffer and more brittle, which may in the long run cause breakage problems. In general, though, henna is an easy way to add body to thin hair.

Q. As I get older and my hair gets lighter, I notice I get a green tinge in it after I swim. What causes that?

A. Many people, mostly blonde, blame the chlorine in swimming pools for that fashionable green look. Actually, they should place the blame on some of the copper-based algicides used in pools. The only thing we can suggest is to shampoo right after swimming or keep the hair short. Try an acidic shampoo and a conditioner. If the hair is still green, a weak solution of hydrogen peroxide may bring it back to normal. There is supposed to be a new product on the market, a preswim treatment to avoid greening of the hair, but we have yet to see it.

Q. This is not for me, of course, but a friend of mine is getting a little older (ahem) and has developed just a few gray, coarse hairs on her face. Is there anything she can do for that?

A. This is a very common phenomenon in older women, probably related to heredity or hormonal changes, and is easy to treat. If you only have a few hairs in the area, electrolysis is fine. It's not 100 percent effective and may be a little uncomfortable. A few hairs will grow back, but you can go back and repeat the procedure. There are few side effects and the removal is permanent. Little dark spots sometimes appear where the hair used to be, but it's very rare. Electrolysis is usually done by a trained practitioner to whom your dermatologist can refer you. There are also machines you can buy for doing your own electrolysis at home. They do work, but they take a certain degree of expertise. Plucking and waxing are also acceptable means of removing hair, though of course they are not permanent. Shaving and depilatories are fine.

Q. Is it possible for gray hair to return to its original color?

A. If hair goes gray as a result of infection, injury, emotional problems, or neurological problems, new hair will often grow back with stronger pigment when the situation is corrected. Hair that turns gray in the natural course of aging is gray forever.

Q. Is waxing safe for removing excess hair on the upper lip and other areas?

A. In the opinion of many, waxing is the best method of removing hair. Heat wax until it softens, then let it cool to a temperature that will not burn the skin. Apply it to the skin, let it dry and harden, and then peel it off against the grain (the angle at which the hair grows out), pulling the hair out by its roots. Clean the area thoroughly with soap and water, dry thoroughly, and apply a bland, nonperfumed emollient. Contrary to popular belief, waxing does not increase coarseness or pigment in the hair. On the upper lip, it need be done only once every four to six weeks.

Q. I'm going to have surgery to remove a growth close to my hairline and I'll have to keep my hair dry for a week. How can I possibly keep my hair clean?

A. There is such a thing as a dry shampoo. It's not as effective as regular shampoo, but it's certainly better than nothing. It removes surface oils and dirt, but is not very good at cleansing the scalp effectively. But, used regularly, it can let you go longer between regular shampoos.

Q. What about estrogen for hair loss?

A. For many years it was thought that estrogens applied locally or taken internally could stop hair loss in women, and at one time this therapy was used almost as a routine. But more recent studies indicate that locally applied estrogen has no effect on hair growth, and internal estrogen therapy rarely helps.

Q. Can women have hair transplants?

A. In women whose thinning hair has become a real cosmetic problem, hair transplants may be one answer. A transplant takes hair from the back or side of the scalp, where hair is thicker, and relocates it in the thinning area. Many women prefer a transplant to continuous use of wigs.

Q. How much does a hair transplant cost?

A. It depends on how much hair is transplanted. Most physicians can, for a fee, provide an initial consultation, at which time they can estimate how much hair would have to be transplanted and how many sessions would be required.

Q. Is it true that if you pull out a gray hair, two will grow back?

A. No. Except in certain disease states, a hair follicle can only grow one hair at a time. If you pull out a gray hair, only one hair will grow back—and it will be gray.

Q. Is there any danger in using hair dryers?

A. Hair dryers are not only time savers, they are, in general, very safe for the hair. In the studies that have been done, hair will usually get oily again more quickly if dried electrically than manually. As far as temperature goes, you would need 150 degrees centigrade before you could damage the keratin in the hair. The dryer would melt long before it got that hot.

FIVE

The Dermatologists' Guide to Beauty Salons

Our stock answer for patients who asked about facials used to go something like this: "We don't think *we* would care for it, but there's nothing wrong with it for the type of person who likes to be pampered and lie around and be waited on."

But that was before Dr. Sternberg *fils* let himself be talked into having a facial at one of Beverly Hills's more stylish salons. This grown man, who usually cannot sit still for a minute, melted into a puddle of relaxation before our very eyes. Whether or not his skin was improved by an avocado mask, low-level ultraviolet light treatment, steaming and cleaning out the pores, and a facial massage we cannot really say. His office assistant said he looked fabulous, but it's only fair to mention she has been lobbying for a raise since 1947. His daughter, on the other hand, asked him the next day when he was going to have his facial. But there was no doubt about the psychological effect. He felt great.

After the facial, we spoke to a number of well-known cosmetologists. Much to our surprise, we came away favorably impressed, not only by their business acumen and personal charm but by their knowledge of dermatology and their basic common sense. They have obviously been learning from the medical profession. Perhaps the medical profession also has something to learn from them.

Naturally, there are things with which we, as dermatologists with a foundation in science, do not agree. Judging by what medicine knows, some of the reasons cosmetologists give for why certain treatments work are, in a word, wrong. But medicine simply has not studied most of the treatments. We have no information one way or the other. Our training and the research of others may tell us that there is no reason for a certain herb to be beneficial. Their experience—and the experience of those who have used such herbs for thousands of years—tells them it works. Who's to say?

In this chapter, we offer our impressions of three beauty salons. We are concerned first with what treatments they offer and what rationales they offer for why those treatments work. Then, from our medical perspective, we discuss the validity of these treatments and rationales.

One enters the Institut de Beauté in Beverly Hills through a large, beautifully decorated wooden-and-leaded-glass door and is instantly thrust into a beehive of activity. Wherever one looks, upstairs or downstairs, people, mostly beautiful, are talking in all languages. But at the center of this beehive, one person is obviously in charge. She holds a reporter from Paris at bay while she conducts a new client into a private room. She scurries from one cosmetologist to another, peeking in on low-lit rooms off a series of corridors with just enough room for one client and the cosmetologist's paraphernalia. The woman has an incredible amount of energy and, just from a brief glimpse, it is easy to see she loves her work. Her name is Aida Grey. She is the daughter of a dermatologist and the author of

THE AIDA GREY BEAUTY BOOK

While the Institut de Beauté offers all sorts of treatments for all sorts of faces, we confined ourselves to questions about the aging skin. She summarized her philosophy of skin care succinctly: "Until age 23, God is responsible for your face. After that, it's your job—and you have the face your deserve." The most important factors in keeping the skin young are, she says, proper cleansing first and foremost, followed by circulation, exercise, disposition, and living right—not necessarily in that order. By exercise, she means exercise of the whole body (presumably for its generally healthful effects), not facial exercise, currently in vogue in some circles. To increase circulation, she recommends a slant board, raising the feet to increase the flow of blood to the head, and even a mild massage or stimulating creams.

Good skin is something one can acquire through education. "I don't believe in miracle creams," she says, "but I do believe in the miracle of habit." Cleansing, stimulating, moisturizing, and lubricating are all extremely important, she says, but there is no fountain of youth. She believes in natural products, made from flowers, herbs, and fruits. Her assortment of masks, some fourteen in all, contains such ingredients as avocado, ginseng, azulene, and aloe vera. She especially likes ginseng, a Chinese herbal root that she says not only softens and tightens wrinkles by increasing the skin's puffiness, but also has a calming effect. But the only kind she finds worthwhile is grown in volcanic soil. She very much dislikes petrolatum and mineral oil in any form. On the subject of buying creams, she had a comment worth repeating: "If you pay $100 for a cream, it should come in a one-gallon jar."

When asked about the cause of wrinkles, she singled out dehydration, abuse of the skin, facial expressions such as frequent squinting and frowning, and the biological process of aging. It was only when we asked specifically about the sun and its effect on wrinkling that she said, "The sun is the worst enemy of the skin," and pointed out that all her products contain the sunscreen PABA. She placed some of the blame for aging on bacteria—specifically bacteria on the skin—sometimes due to pollution in large cities, which can result in enlarged pores, more free fatty acids, and soil on the skin that keeps it from breathing freely.

We like Aida Grey's overall approach to the skin very much, though we would take exception to the emphasis she places on some aspects. We offer the following analysis not as criticism, for we found her a very gracious and knowledgeable person, but for the education of our readers. It is our understanding that dehydration does not *cause* wrinkles, but it certainly makes them more noticeable. The main cause of wrinkles, as we have been repeating throughout this book, is the cumulative effect of ultraviolet light damage to the skin. Everything else adds to it, but compared to UVL is minor. Small, fine wrinkles certainly do become less noticeable when the skin is stretched by absorbing moisture. Aida feels this can be done with foundation; she does not believe in moisturizers for everyday treatment except for damaged or dry skin. We would add, though, that if moisture in the skin is important, it is also important to have some kind of moisturizer to hold the moisture in.

As for the concept of bacteria on the skin contributing to aging, here we must take exception. There is no question that bacteria *inside* the pores and the sebaceous glands play a role in plugging up oil glands and causing whiteheads and blackheads, e.g. acne. But we do not believe that bacteria itself—or free fatty acids, or soil *on* the face—has anything to do with wrinkling. And we do not believe that bacteria from the environment causes large pores. The cleansing procedure she suggests to rid the skin of bacteria, however, does have a beneficial effect—it aids the skin's natural process of shedding dead skin cells and helps smooth the surface.

We must also question whether cosmetics can contain substances to stimulate the skin. If by "stimulation" she means stimulating some vital process such as the activity of the organs, we doubt very much that any of these products stimulate the skin. They may have some effect on the surface of the skin; in fact, the Appendix lists a number of these ingredients and describes the effects claimed for them. But, as we mentioned, there is no medical evidence to suggest that ginseng, for instance, relieves pain or irritation.

We have heard the notion that the skin "breathes" from a number of cosmetologists, and it sent us back to our books to discover whether it actually does or not. As it turns out, the skin *does* breathe slightly; that is, it takes in oxygen and it discharges carbon dioxide. But the amount of "breathing" that goes on is not very significant. The skin loses between 60 and 600 ml of carbon dioxide per hour, about 1 percent of the carbon dioxide released by the lungs in that time. Is that enough to play a role in the maintenance of the skin? If the oxygen does reach the blood underlying the skin, the blood could conceivably become more oxygenated and thus make the skin look rosier. But it's certainly not a crucial part of breathing.

For clients contemplating surgical cosmetic procedures, Aida recommends special treatment starting a month before the procedures to learn how to take care of the skin post-op and how to use makeup. For the redness, soreness, and inflammation that sometimes accompany chemical peels, she uses masks of azulene and aloe vera. She claims the masks hasten healing. Though plastic surgeons often recommend using Crisco™ or Vaseline® after a peel, she claims they cause whiteheads and/or milia. Rub some aloe vera or a broken-open capsule of Vitamin E on the face, she says, and you won't get any whiteheads. Though one of her fourteen masks contains collagen, she does not think much of collagen in general. She does not claim it retards aging but does think it improves the skin's surface condition. Despite the recent new developments in injectable collagen, she still prefers silicone and tells us that, in the Orient, beauty salons have been injecting silicone for years.

Aloe vera has been used for many years on minor burns, so perhaps it makes sense to use it after chemical peels. But, since it's made up of about 99 percent water (the rest being carbohydrates and amino acids) it's quite possible that the water accounts for all the soothing effect. If Crisco or Vaseline were really the cause of milia, one would assume everybody would get milia after using them, but in fact milia are rather rare. (Milia are small white "cysts" about one or two millimeters in diameter which occasionally occur a month or two after a chemical peel.) We don't think they are caused by these products. Whether Crisco or Vaseline are the best products to use is another question. We are definitely against using Vitamin E after a peel. We have seen a number of allergic reactions to Vitamin E when used topically and the last thing you want on freshly peeled skin is an allergic reaction, which can increase the depth of destruction produced by the peel and lead to possible scarring. We agree that topical collagen has no permanent effect on the aging process. Topical collagen cream is only as good as the cream itself. In fact, some creams might be more effective, and surely less expensive, *without* the collagen. However, the collagen can form a semipermeable barrier on the skin which retards evaporation of natural moisture. We will discuss silicone, peels, and collagen in later chapters.

Aida Grey is the first to admit her treatments are not panaceas. They are just temporary. But we think she is honest and well informed and that her treatments, performed regularly, correctly, and with the right materials, can help you maintain a soft, better-looking skin.

Sofia Katzman, a cosmetologist and esthetician in Westwood, California, offers a different approach to many of the same concepts. Trained in Poland where she spent the required three years at an institute managed by dermatologists (in her case, two who are well known in American medical circles via their writing), Sofia specializes in facials and electrolysis. She uses herbal masks and uses the same kind of pore cleansing we use in our office. When we do it, we call it acne surgery.

Like Aida Grey, she does not put the major blame for aging on the sun. She points instead to psychological problems, relaxation, and diet. Like Aida Grey, she uses herbal masks, but some of hers get quite exotic—for instance a "Japan mask" made from the yolks of quail eggs and a "king's mask" made from the milk of the queen bee. In evaluating these masks, we are still faced with the same problem: we have no evidence that these ingredients work, but her experience says they do.

Sofia sees her clients about once a month for deep pore cleansing and a facial. She has them supplement the office care with a home treatment emphasizing soap, water, a light cream if necessary, and occasionally cleansing grains for deeper home cleansing. Her facials last fifteen to twenty minutes, during which time a small electrical apparatus keeps the substance warm for increased softness and moisturizing. For her deep pore cleansing, which she believes essential for allowing the skin to breathe, she uses the same instrument dermatologists use for treating whiteheads and blackheads. She believes, and we agree, that some medical training is essential to proper use of this procedure. Improper massage can increase the damage to already sun-damaged skin.

The atmosphere at Aida Thibiant's skin and body care salon on Cañon Drive in Beverly Hills is just the opposite of that at Aida Grey's Institut de Beauté a few blocks away. One is immediately struck by the quiet serenity of the salon. Here no one runs around. There are no loud noises. No one talks. From the front door, relaxation pervades the air and low, indirect lighting in the private rooms enhances the feeling. We have acne to thank for the Aida Thibiant salon; as a young woman she was so impressed by what proper skin care could do for her bad case of acne that she resolved to go into the business herself. She studied at four or five different schools in Paris—not, like some students we know, because she was asked to leave, but because she wanted to be exposed to a variety of styles and techniques.

A woman reaches her peak at age twenty-eight, says Aida Thibiant; from there, it's all downhill. Once the damage is done, we would agree with her that surgery is the best answer. But short of that, she offers a number of temporary treatments. In her own line of cosmetics, she seems particularly concerned that they be as close as possible to hypoallergenic. She does not like lanolin because of its high incidence of allergic reaction. Though she acknowledges the danger of sun damage to aging skin, she omits PABA from all of her products except one, because of PABA allergy reports in some people. This makes sense to us. If you put PABA in all your products, anyone who is allergic to PABA cannot use them. If you offer one that contains PABA, those who want PABA can use that product or any of the others if they combine it with PABA from another source. She does not like mineral oils because they stay on the upper layer of the skin and clog it instead of penetrating. She does not like waxes, because they are heavy, or heavy creams around the eyes at night, which can clog up pores and, she feels, may actually *cause* baggy eyes in the morning. She believes in light creams—even though many people distrust something they can barely feel. Actually, light creams that soak in are the best for moisturizing, she says. There is no question that heavy oils on the face can cause cosmetic problems like clogged pores *(acne cosmetica)*. And we like her attitude about new wonder cosmetics like collagen and jojoba—we cannot know what they do until they have been used and tested a lot longer.

Deep pore cleansing in her salon is done manually, using the fingers and gauze or cloth. This can be beneficial —if done correctly. Pores free of dried oil plugs enable the oil to flow freely as it should so that oil glands do not enlarge and become noticeable. Of course, the plugs go right ahead and form again after the cleansing. And if done incorrectly, pore cleansing can rupture the oil glands beneath the skin, resulting in inflammation.

Throwing caution to the wind, we ventured to ask what she thought of the advice dermatologists generally give their patients about skin care. Too much drying, she said. They almost always recommend drying out the skin, especially for acne or oily skin. In the long run, she says, drying can make matters worse. We cannot disagree with that. Dermatologists do try to dry the skin, though that is changing in the treatment of acne. Modern acne research leads us to say which soap you use is not as important as how you use it. Overvigorous cleansing should not break the pimples. Vigorous washing with detergents, five or six times a day, brings on an acne with a name all its own, *acne detergi-*

cans. Another criticism she had of dermatologists is that they do not spend enough time with their patients, and we cannot argue with that either. Many dermatologists are enthusiastic about explaining things when they first start out, but as they get older and busier and find themselves saying the same things over and over, they tend to get lax about it. Patient education is extremely important—especially in convincing a patient to stick to a new regimen. Most dermatological treatments take time to work, and a patient who understands the goals and procedures will be a patient patient.

We come now to the *pièce de résistance*—Dr. Sternberg's facial. It started with deep pore cleansing. His assistant, looking on appreciatively, said it was just as good as what she does in the office. Then a substance known by the clinical name of "green goop" was applied to his face. In order to make it penetrate the skin better, he was given an electrode to hold in his hand while an instrument emitting galvanic current massaged the goop into his face. The theory was that the molecules in the goop would ionize and be drawn into the skin by the electrical current. That may or may not work, but it sounds good and whether it worked or not it was relaxing. Next came a cooling cream, whose prime ingredient we could easily identify from the smell—camphor. After that, the cosmetologist pulled out something that looked like an electric toothbrush with the stem and base of a wine glass instead of a brush. When she turned it on, it flashed blue—high-frequency-current ultraviolet light, she said, claiming it kills bacteria and can clear up a pimple overnight. We have our doubts about that one. If it gives out enough ultraviolet light to do anything like that, it gives out enough to cause damage. Not even the sun's UVL can clear up pimples overnight. It does have a nice psychological effect, but if it does anything more than that we surely don't know why.

The facial concluded with a light massage. Says Dr. Sternberg, "When it was all done, I can honestly say that I was very relaxed and stayed relaxed for the rest of the day. And I could feel the difference on my face. My skin felt just a little bit of a tingle to it, just a little bit tighter." The tightening may be due to the combination of moisture and the herbs drying on the skin. Camphor, with its mild anesthetic effect, could account for the tingling. And the reviews of his appearance, as we mentioned earlier, were mixed— though, he confesses, he did none of the follow-up care strongly recommended.

We think the psychological aspect plays a big role in the effectiveness of facials. When you relax, your features relax. When your features relax, you look younger. After an hour of lying on one's back in a comfortable room with soft light, being massaged and talked to by a pleasant person, getting steam and soothing face masks, who wouldn't feel and look better? Aida Thibiant admits that the psychotherapeutic aspect accounts for 50 percent of the facial's success.

After meeting these cosmetologists, we have new respect for the business. If the cosmetologist knows what he or she is doing and uses the correct procedures, a facial *can* help the skin's appearance. It will hurt nothing but your wallet.

QUESTIONS AND ANSWERS

Q. Is it true that bacteria on the skin play a role in its appearance? What protection does the skin have against bacteria?

A. The skin protects itself in many ways. First is "desquamation" or sloughing off of the skin, i.e. the outer skin cells, which goes on all the time. Hundreds of thousands of microorganisms come off with the cells as the skin desquamates. Second is the effect of natural dessication or drying. Many bacteria cannot live in a dry environment. Third is antimicrobial chemicals found on the skin, like free fatty acids—the ones everybody is so worried about removing. In fact, free fatty acids cause the low pH of the skin, which is around 5.5. The normally acidic skin has an antibiotic or antimicrobial effect. It may be interesting to note that the reason these free fatty acids exist on the skin is that microorganisms feeding on the lipids of the skin break them down into free fatty acids, which, being acid, then result in the demise of the same microorganisms that created them in the first place. In other words, it's sort of an unintentional suicide. They dig their own graves by what they eat. Fourth, we harbor a lot of microorganisms that are antagonistic to one another, which, in an ecological niche, keeps the numbers down. All of these things tend to decrease the amount of bacteria on the skin and decrease the possibility of infection.

Q. Do mudpacks do anything for the skin?

A. A clay or mudpack or any of the packs that dry the skin is designed to pick up oil from oily skin, to pick up cellular debris, to make the skin smoother, and to result in a tightening of the skin which makes those very fine wrinkles, at least temporarily, less noticeable.

Q. What do you think about lanolin in cosmetics?

A. Lanolin is a natural product, obtained from the fleece of sheep, and it varies in its constituents from time to time. We do not know exactly why it is allergenic, but it is one of the more important causes of what we call cutaneous sensitization. People who are allergic to one kind of lanolin preparation may be able to tolerate another preparation quite well. You could conceivably be allergic to lanolin alcohol but be completely unallergic to lanolin sterol. In certain susceptible people, lanolin can cause whiteheads and blackheads.

Q. Do you think I should have a facial?

A. It depends on what kind of facial you have and for what reason. There are many varieties. Done for the right reasons and by well-trained practitioners, a facial will cause no harm and is often beneficial.

SIX

Face Peels

There is nothing new about peeling the upper layer of the skin in order to get at healthier or more attractive skin below. Ancient Egyptian documents written on papyrus describe recipes for smoothing the skin and removing blemishes. The Egyptians used alabaster, pumice, salt, and extracts of animal oil; modern Americans still use pumice, mixed with almond grit for beauty creams or replaced by polyethylene granules for abrasive soaps. But the best peels we can offer today involve chemicals such as resorcin, salicylic acid, and the two most popular—phenol and trichloroacetic acid (TCA).

Whichever chemical is used, the basic goal is the same. First, the chemical destroys the epidermis and the uppermost part of the dermis. Then, as the skin heals from below, the new skin shows less sun damage, pigmentation, and signs of age, and fewer freckles and fine wrinkles.

Chemical face peels have been used for many years—phenol (also known as carbolic acid) since the 1950s—but it was not until the medical profession started looking at them closely, in the 1960s, that they became the refined treatments they are today. Earlier, their use had been primarily confined to cosmetologists and the results were inconsistent. Now, in the best examples, chemical face peels can produce a smoothness of skin that a facelift alone cannot.

The ideal patient for a chemical peel is a thin-skinned female with fair complexion, light eyes, and fine wrinkles. If laxity and/or sagging of the skin is also a problem, chemical peels can supplement other procedures, like facelifts. Chemical peels have been used with good results for treating multiple solar keratoses and other sun damage and for treating irregular or spotty increases in pigmentation. They have been used with fair to good results for treating certain kinds of superficial acne scars.

Be forewarned, though, that chemical peels can involve several weeks of discomfort and a change in appearance that gets worse before it gets better. It cannot be overemphasized that the right mental preparation for a face peel requires a complete understanding of what's to come. Since everyone's self-image and tolerance for pain is different, only consultation with an experienced physician and with other people who have undergone the procedure can give you a sufficient idea in advance. (And keep in mind that your friends may be more or less sensitive to pain and self-image than you are.) In this chapter, we attempt to provide some of that crucial understanding.

HOW A FACE PEEL WORKS

A chemical face peel starts by deliberately damaging the skin. It creates a controlled wound similar to a second-degree burn. A first-degree burn, as you may know, is fairly mild—about the severity of a bad sunburn. A third-degree burn is the worst—it goes deep, wiping out nerves and skin structure, refusing to heal, and often requiring skin grafts. A second-degree burn, then, is somewhere in the middle. It burns down deep into the dermis and, since it does not destroy nerve endings, is initially more painful than a third-degree burn. It leaves skin structures, such as hair follicles and oil glands, intact.

As the peeling substance removes the entire epidermis and a portion of the dermis, oozing from underlying tissue and crust formation begins. It is not, as one might expect, a question of cells starting to grow back. Rather, cells from around the edge of the wound start moving in to fill in the wound and cells from the remaining structures that lie in the deeper layers of the skin move up. When they meet, having filled in the wound, this migration of cells stops. It is not until two or three days after the peel that new cells start to form, but that initial migration of neighboring cells starts as early as eighteen hours after the peel. Until the new cells begin to grow, the area is still thin, and thus, more sensitive to chemicals. For that reason, you will be asked to keep medicated cosmetics, vitamins, and the like off the skin during this period.

The underlying dermis takes longer to heal than the surface epidermis. New collagen forms, sometimes in horizontal lines parallel to the surface of the skin instead of the random pattern found in the undamaged dermis. It is this new collagen that is responsible for any improvement in wrinkles or texture that may follow the peel.

THE PROCEDURE—PHENOL

A face peel can be applied to the entire face or to just one region, perhaps the "purse-string" wrinkles around the mouth. It can be done in the hospital or the doctor's office, with or without general anesthesia. Whether or not a full face peel is done in the hospital may depend on whether the masking that follows the application of the chemical is done with waterproof tape or ointment. Many physicians recommend that a full face peel with tape be done only in the hospital.

The most widely used phenol mixture is a precise combination of phenol, Croton oil, distilled water, and liquified soap. (We do not give the exact formula because we do not want to encourage misunderstandings: this is *not* a home procedure.) Phenol causes an immediate breakdown of cells, followed by coagulation. Used as more than 80 percent of the mixture, it causes enough coagulation to prevent penetration beyond a certain depth. The Croton oil, also an irritant, helps the phenol destroy the epidermis more rapidly and penetrate more deeply into the dermal layer. Tape or ointment masking keeps the peeling agent from evaporating and this prolongs the chemical action.

If you have a prior history of sensitivity to phenol or have had a previous phenol peel, your treatment may start with a test peel, usually of a small area in front of the ear, to make sure you will not react adversely to the peeling agent. Once cleared, you will have your face well-cleansed the night before and again with acetone or ether just before starting the procedure to remove all residual oil. Medication for relaxation and to decrease pain will be administered at this time.

For a full facial peel, the physician starts by dividing the face into sections and applying the phenol to each section separately. For a regional peel, he uses a "feathering" technique. This spreads the substance into natural facial divisions without causing lines of demarcation between the peeled and nonpeeled areas. A white frost will appear on the face when the phenol reaction begins. It is accompanied by a burning, painful sensation that usually lasts ten to fifteen seconds and can be quite uncomfortable. It recurs in five to twenty minutes and may last, in varying degrees, for seven to ten days. Sometimes itching can occur. As the physician finishes each section, he tapes it and moves on to the next. Slow application is the best way to avoid complications associated with the skin's absorption of phenol.

The tape stays on for forty-eight hours; the patient stays sedated during this time and should have easy access to medication for any associated pain. Food is limited to fluid through a straw and talking should be kept to a minimum. At the end of the forty-eight hours, after more pain medication, the tape is removed to reveal a raw, moist face. For three days, the face is treated with either a Thymol iodide powder or an antibiotic-based powder two or three times a day. After five days, the patient can switch to a bland cold cream or antibiotic ointment. On the sixth day, the crusted powder mask that has built up from the application of these materials comes off—to reveal an intensely pink new skin. The intensity fades, after a week of moisturizing creams, to a persistent redness or erythema. At this point, a light makeup (preferably water-based, because it is the easiest to remove) is permitted, to be replaced by regular makeup in two to three weeks.

Taping or masking generally makes for a deeper peel and protects the skin against inadvertent scratching, which can result in scars. There is, however, some debate about the merits of taping. A deeper peel carries an increased risk of complication and we now know that immediate and continuous use of an occlusive ointment, directly following the phenol application, can give gratifying results while eliminating the need for hospitalization and a second anesthetic and/or analgesic. Use of ointment is also more convenient and comfortable for the patient. Why would any one want a tape peel, then? Simply because the debate is not yet resolved and there are still those who believe that tape gives a better result. We recommend leaving the decision up to the physician, based on his experience and his estimate of what would be best for you. In order to do that comfortably, one must have a trusting patient-physician relationship.

After a nontape peel, the patient can go home as soon as the vital signs are stable and there is no sign of complications—usually two to four hours after the procedure. A continuous film is kept, usually an antibiotic ointment, on the face for three days and washing the face is not allowed. An internal broad-spectrum antibiotic will be taken during this time and the face should be fully covered with ointment —at all times. For the first three days, the physician will examine the results often. After this period, the face can be washed two or three times a day with a mild soap and lukewarm water. If there is any discomfort or any signs of continued peeling, a moisturizing cream can be used. At the end of a week, the skin will be about as pink as it would be with a tape peel, and the healing process from then on is quite similar. Within seven to ten days, the patient can go back to work.

COMPLICATIONS

Phenol face peels have some very real and potentially dangerous side effects. We believe, however, that chemical peeling is a safe and effective procedure when performed correctly. The most serious possible side effect of phenol peeling results from systemic absorption of phenol. Phenol poisoning can lead to depression of the central nervous system, which can show up as decreased temperature, coma, cardiac irregularity, and respiratory arrest. Patients have died from phenol peels. Phenol is poisonous to the heart and, since it is excreted via the kidneys, can also damage the kidneys. If too large an area is treated too rapidly, heart irregularities may result. We minimize these systemic problems by the kind of section-by-section application described previously under "The Procedure."

The most common complications have to do with pigmentation. Skin that regrows in peeled areas is usually lighter and smoother than the surrounding skin. While this is usually considered an improvement and referred to as "the alabaster look," it can call attention to itself if the untreated skin surrounding the area is in great contrast. For that reason, we use the "feathering" or blending technique described above and try to extend the peel into the hairline and onto the lip to keep the demarcation to a minimum. Against the permanently lighter skin in the peeled area, pigmented moles that did not call attention before may now stand out more. On rare occasions, peeled areas heal darker or hyperpigmented, although this is a more common complication with more superficial peels. Those with dark or olive skin and an oily complexion may experience mottled, irregular pigmentation. If it does occur, it can sometimes—but, unfortunately, not always—be treated by repeating the peel without tape masking three months later. Since pregnancy, oral contraceptives, and exposure to the sun affect pigmentation, they should be avoided for at least six months after the procedure is completed. Persistent redness lasts six to twelve weeks; beyond that, it can be treated.

Scarring, a rare side effect, has been reported on the jawline and neck and, to a lesser degree, on the upper and lower eyelids. To minimize the possibility of scarring, these areas should not be taped. Anything that produces pressure on the peeled area, such as a shower cap or a head band, should be avoided, since the pressure could turn the desired second-degree wound into a third-degree wound and third-degree wounds leave scars.

Milia—to repeat, are small white "cysts" about one to two millimeters in diameter—occasionally occur a month or two after a chemical peel. If they persist, a physician can "uncap" them or they can be treated with very gentle use of a mild abrasive.

Cold sores or fever blisters often break out four to seven days after the peel in patients with a history of herpetic infections on the lips or face. These people should make sure that their physician knows about their medical history. The outbreak can be treated with antiviral medication.

It may come as a surprise to learn that infection is one of the least common complications, but not if one considers the meticulous cleansing of the skin that precedes the treatment, the ability of the peeling agent to kill bacteria, and the antibiotics that are part of the treatment.

Though we have listed a number of unpleasant complications, it must be remembered that, for the most part, they can be controlled by careful use of the proper technique and materials. The deep phenol peel is an excellent treatment, either alone or in combination with other plastic procedures, for the treatment of wrinkles.

TRICHLOROACETIC ACID PEELS (TCA)

Trichloroacetic acid (TCA) has been used for many years in various concentrations.

Fifteen–20 percent, the lightest TCA peel, results in a very light scaling of the uppermost part of the epidermis and is most often used for areas of increased pigment such as chloasma (mask of pregnancy) or the similar melasma, often a complication of oral contraceptives. The 15–20 percent solution has little long-term effect on wrinkles.

Preparation for the 15–20 percent TCA peel is very similar to that of the phenol peel, involving a careful cleansing of the face. As the TCA is applied very smoothly to the skin, the skin turns white and there is a bit of stinging. Premedication is not usually necessary, but can be used at the discretion of the physician. Isopropyl alcohol followed by ice packs with mild pressure neutralize the

TCA and decrease swelling. Within three to five minutes the stinging stops and the patient feels a persistent tightness of the face but little pain. In two to three days, the face peels, getting very dry and itchy. For itching and redness, a 1 percent hydrocortisone lotion can be used.

The peeling is similar to what happens after a sunburn. Don't pull off the loose edges, though; you may pull off an area that is not yet ready to come off and cause deeper damage. You may, however, snip off the ends with scissors to keep the face smooth. The irritation of the chemical peel causes a mild swelling, which tends to make wrinkles less noticeable. We must caution, though, that this is not a treatment for wrinkles. As soon as the swelling is gone, the wrinkles will be back. It takes five to ten days for your face to heal completely, so you can be back at work within a week.

Twenty-five–35 percent TCA gives a little deeper peel used to treat sun-damaged skin with keratoses—the sun-weathered skin common at the end of the summer. It is not a long-term treatment for wrinkles. The procedure is the same as for the 20 percent peel, except that, since the 25–35 percent peel is a deeper peel, it naturally takes a little longer to heal.

Fifty percent TCA is probably the weakest solution that can have a long-term effect on wrinkles. It does not give as deep a peel as phenol, but it does usually result in a noticeable improvement and carries less risk of side effects. (It should be noted again that side effects with phenol are also rare.) Preparation and procedure are the same except that, since the 50 percent peel is deeper and, thus, less comfortable, the patient is premedicated and given an antibiotic ointment after treatment. It takes longer to heal—about ten days to two weeks—and the pinkness persists a bit longer. The patient can go back to work two weeks after the procedure is performed.

The 50 percent peel is used for the treatment of freckles and fine wrinkles. It is rarely used with tape or masking. The 100 percent peel, which approaches phenol in its depth of destruction, is also rarely used.

The neck can also be treated with TCA, but there are many problems involved. It may be because the skin of the neck is thinner or because it contains fewer supporting structures such as oil glands and hair follicles. Whatever the reason, there are more complications; enough that some physicians prefer not to treat the neck at all. When the neck *is* treated, thirty-five percent is the strongest solution that can be used.

COMPLICATIONS

To our knowledge, there have been no deaths reported with the use of TCA. It is not toxic to the heart or kidneys, but there are other possible complications. The most common are increased pigmentation, which tends to fade by itself or can be treated with bleach creams, and decreased pigmentation, a much less common complication more often seen with the stronger solutions. Infection can occur despite the use of antibiotic ointments, but if recognized early can be easily treated and does not result in permanent damage. Untreated, infection can result in scarring, a rare but occasionally reported side effect.

The swelling might technically be considered a complication, but it has the positive effect of stretching and plumping out the skin, thus making the wrinkles less noticeable. Again, the wrinkles are not really gone. But they may appear to be gone until the swelling subsides.

In general, the weaker the solution, the smaller the chance there is of complications. But, as we like to mention from time to time, everyone is different. Even the skin on the same face is different from section to section. What may be a weak solution may have a strong effect from section to section or individual to individual.

QUESTIONS AND ANSWERS

Q. What does a peel cost?

A. A quick check of doctors' offices in the Los Angeles area surprised us. The same procedure done by reputable physicians, any of whom we could recommend with confidence, can vary widely in price. A phenol peel done by a plastic surgeon ranges from $300 when done with a facelift, to $500 and as much as $1,200 for a full face. A TCA peel ranges from $250 for a partial peel with a 25 percent solution to $500 for a full face using 25 percent to anywhere from $600 to $1,500 for a full face using 50 percent. A partial dermabrasion goes for $500; a full face dermabrasion anywhere from $1,200 to $2,500 for the same treatment.

Q. I've heard that many cosmetic or plastic surgeons require payment in advance instead of after the operation. Why is this?

A. Since cosmetic surgery is elective surgery it is not covered by insurance. The procedure is usually expensive and takes a great deal of the surgeon's time. So, to avoid the regrettable but common problem of delinquent accounts, they charge in advance.

Q. Will my health insurance cover cosmetic surgery?

A. Since we have not read your insurance policy, we cannot say for sure, but in most cases insurance only covers reconstructive surgery to correct a medical problem or a disfigurement caused by trauma, accident, or birth. While you may argue that your big nose is a disfigurement caused by birth (and causing great trauma), few insurance companies are likely to agree.

Q. Does the age at which you have an initial face peel or dermabrasion have any relationship to the length of time the results will last?

A. The younger you are, the less your tissues have been damaged and the better you heal. If you have such a treatment at an early age and then go on a very rigid program of skin care and protection from the sun, it would seem reasonable to assume that the results would last longer and be more satisfactory. However, we are talking about a cosmetic procedure—and generally you would want to wait until you feel it's really necessary.

Q. Are there wrong reasons to have cosmetic treatments?

A. Absolutely—and physicians keep a careful eye out for them. A patient may have an insignificant deformity which becomes, in his or her mind, the cause of all problems. "If only I had a face peel, then people would like me and I could get a job and be more popular." Chances are this is not so. Chemical peels come from a doctor's office, not an employment bureau. Surgery cannot change behavior or make social problems disappear. It can only change the way you look, and even that is limited by what kind of structure you have beneath the skin. On the other hand, if you understand the possibilities and limitations of a procedure realistically and correcting an image problem will make you feel better and you have the money to spend, there's no reason not to go ahead with it.

Q. How will I look after a peel?

A. Experienced physicians can make predictions, but there are no guarantees, simply because there are too many variables. Do you tend to bleed, scar, or pigment? How well do you heal? How well do you resist infection? What is your age and general health? There's also something called luck.

You could be a perfect candidate with the perfect doctor and get the performance of the doctor's career only to walk out the office, trip on the sidewalk, and scratch your face, leaving a permanent scar.

Q. Can I die from a cosmetic procedure?

A. Anything is possible, but it is highly unlikely. People who have cosmetic or elective surgery are generally in good health. It's not an emergency. It's done under the best of conditions. There's a small risk associated with use of anesthesia and, of course, there's always the possibility of a drug reaction. But these things are very, very rare.

Q. What if I'm dissatisfied with the results of the procedure?

A. The most common mistake people make is to expect instant beauty. It's really not fair to judge the results right after having the procedure. Swelling and discoloration may not completely subside for three to six months. But if, after a reasonable wait, you are still dissatisfied you are entitled to confront the physician. If he agrees with you, he may well recommend doing another procedure and may not charge you. If he does not agree with you and feels that it *is,* in fact, a good result, you can always get a second opinion.

Q. What about these polyester sponges and other ways of peeling the skin at home?

A. Synthetic polyester sponges or mechanical abraders like luffa, available in most drug stores, have long been used to peel the skin, but it's only recently that good studies have been done. The "peel" of this type makes the surface of the skin smoother and more regular which in turn makes the skin easier to clean. By removing the drier, superficial cells that have yet to slough off by themselves, it becomes easier to keep the skin moisturized. This method has its place, but it should not be abused. The present feeling is that it should not be used on normal skin because it is very drying.

Q. If a face peel is similar to a second degree burn, why is there no scarring?

A. Scarring occurs when a wound is deep and severe, enough to wipe out all the existing adnexal structures—that is, sweat glands, oil glands, hair follicles, and the rest. Since healing originates with these structures, it is only when you go deep enough to destroy them that scarring occurs.

Q. Why would anyone want to have a facelift and *a chemical peel?*

A. Facelifts can get rid of sagging tissues and stretch certain areas of the skin. This helps get rid of certain wrinkles, especially the deeper ones. But facelifts do not generally affect the wrinkles found on the upper lip, forehead, and eyelids. These can benefit from a chemical peel.

Q. If I have a face peel, when should I expect to see results?

A. You'll see the immediate results after the first six to twelve weeks—a decrease in the amount of fine wrinkles, due to the swelling, and a persistent redness or pinkness. It will be four or five months, when deeper tissues like the dermis and the collagen can replace and/or heal themselves, until you see the maximum benefits.

Q. I had an entire face peel done about three years ago and just recently have noticed some new fine wrinkles around the mouth. Do I need another complete peel?

A. Just because you've had a complete face peel before does not mean you have to treat the entire face each time. Local touch-ups may be done as needed.

Q. What are facial peels best at?

A. Facial peels have their best results with fine wrinkling and spotty hyperpigmentation (local areas of darker skin color).

Q. Why is the skin color lighter after a chemical peel and what does it mean?

A. Apparently chemical peels remove a significant amount of the melanin-producing cells (melanocytes) in the basal layer of the epidermis. Naturally, with a reduction in the number of pigment-making cells, you get not only a lighter skin color but less protection against the sun.

Q. Are chemical peels any good for small broken blood vessels and capillaries on the face?

A. Sometimes a patient shows some improvement, but not usually. Peeling is not recommended for treatment of broken blood vessels.

Q. I had a phenol face peel and subsequently developed an allergic reaction. Are there any other things that I should watch out for?

A. Phenol or carbolic acid is a coal tar derivative. There are certain substances that it *may,* and we underline the word may, cross-react with. A certain number of people who are allergic to phenol also develop an allergic reaction when they come in contact with resorcin and resorcinols or hydroquinone. Resorcin and resorcinols are found in antidandruff shampoos and are sometimes used in hair dyes, lipsticks, hair tonics, scalp lotions, and acne preparations. They should be listed on the label. Hydroquinone is a common ingredient in bleach or "freckle" creams; in fact, it is the active ingredient, bringing about the lightening of the skin. Cresols, used in hair preparations and some eye lotions as antiseptics and disinfectants, can also cross-react.

Q. Are chemical peels a treatment for enlarged pores?

A. No they are not, though we are frequently asked if they are. In fact, some patients think their pores actually increase in size after the peel. Probably the pores have not increased in size—they are just more obvious now because the wrinkles are less noticeable.

Q. How long does a phenol peel last?

A. In general, one to five years.

Q. Who does phenol peels?

A. Generally speaking, phenol peels are done by plastic surgeons, while TCA is more in the realm of dermatologists. Naturally there are exceptions.

SEVEN

5-Fluorouracil and Other Treatments for Damaged Skin

Wrinkles and sagging are the most common manifestations of aging skin. But solar keratoses—those hard, scaly, red lesions that occur conspicuously and in various sizes on sun-exposed skin—can make a convincing claim for second place. Nature continues to pick on the fair-skinned person who spends or misspends his or her youth in the great outdoors. Solar keratoses can be quite unattractive, particularly as they can occur in large quantities, and are considered to be premalignant. Left untreated, 20 to 25 percent of them will very slowly turn into skin cancer.

Fortunately, there are several ways of treating solar keratoses. These include:

- Freezing with liquid nitrogen (LN_2) or carbon dioxide (CO_2), also known as cryotherapy
- Scraping with a curette
- Electrodessication plus scraping with a curette

- Trichloroacetic acid or phenol applications
- 5-Fluorouracil peels

We will examine each of these treatments in detail, but first let us answer the most important question. How do you know if you have solar keratoses? Solar keratoses start off as smooth, brownish-red spots similar to liver spots *(lentigines)*. The difference is that solar keratoses continue to progress. They become raised and feel scratchy to the touch, as if you were running your finger over a fine grade of sandpaper. Left untreated, they become even more raised, often developing a thick keratin plug in the middle that makes the whole thing look like a miniature volcano. In the case of a particularly long plug, the formation goes by the unappetizing name "cutaneous horn." Because of their relation to sun damage, keratoses are found most often on the arms, hands, and face and only rarely in areas that are usually covered by clothing.

Solar keratoses can give the skin an aged look far beyond its years—but they can be treated. Since the damage is due to ultraviolet light damage, which is cumulative and irreversible, there is no way to eliminate the problem entirely. Some kind of treatment will be necessary for the rest of your life, ranging from one or two office visits per year for a mild case to monthly visits for a severe case. But the treatments *can* catch keratoses before they become cancerous. And their removal will make the skin look younger.

CRYOTHERAPY

For treatment of a small number of keratoses, our first choice is liquid nitrogen. It is quick and effective, does not result in scarring (in rare cases, a white spot will be left at the treatment site), and it is relatively inexpensive—especially since, for insurance purposes, it is considered a substitute for surgery.

In our office we apply liquid nitrogen with copper-tipped instruments that, when placed in the liquid nitrogen, assume its temperature—minus 196 degrees centigrade. When the applicator first touches your skin, you may feel a sensation of heat, which is actually, of course, extreme cold. The applicator, applied with moderate pressure for four to ten seconds depending on how thick the keratosis is, freezes the skin and turns it white, deadening the nerves. When the applicator is removed and the skin thaws, there is a stinging sensation for one to five minutes, but little discomfort after that.

Over the next twenty-four to forty-eight hours, a scab and, on rare occasions, a blister may form. On even rarer occasions, a blood blister may form. Pressure from the fluid inside the blister may cause pain—so it is all right to pop the blister and relieve the pressure. Clean the blister first with rubbing or isopropyl alcohol. Then, with a sterile instrument such as a pin that has been held under a flame, prick the lower edge of the blister. Scabs last a week, though it will take four weeks for the skin to regenerate. If lesions persist after four weeks, they should be treated again, perhaps with freezing, perhaps with a different approach, and a biopsy may be in order.

Carbon dioxide, at minus 60 degrees centigrade, can accomplish the same result, though it is not as easy to use as liquid nitrogen. Since each application requires its own carbon dioxide gas cartridge, the procedure takes more time and the apparatus is more cumbersome. For that reason, carbon dioxide is now used by very few physicians.

Some patients confess to us that they buy their own dry ice, use some kind of insulating material to hold it, and treat their own keratoses at home. We do not advocate do-it-yourself cryotherapy, but those who insist on it will probably not do themselves harm—unless, being the amateur physicians they are, they have misdiagnosed the case. What if their supposed keratosis is really a spot of eczema or a skin cancer? In that case, it will not respond to the cryotherapy and, unless it responds just like other lesions that have been treated by the physician, it should be immediately brought to the attention of the physician to rule out the possibility of other diseases, especially skin cancer.

ELECTRODESSICATION AND CURETTAGE

For keratoses that do not respond to freezing and for very thick keratoses, the treatment of choice is electrodessication with curettage. After an injection of the anesthetic Xylocaine®, the area is dessicated lightly with an electric needle. Then, using a curette, the physician scrapes off the offending lesion. The advantage is that the scraping provides a biopsy specimen for a skin cancer test. The disadvantage is that it takes longer for a scab to form and the skin to heal with electrodessication than with cryotherapy—and electrodessication leaves a scar. What kind of scar it leaves depends on a number of things: how large the lesion was, how deep it went, where on the body it was located, or how well the patient heals. It can range from a white spot with very little depression in a fair-skinned person to a keloid in people prone to developing keloids. (The keloid, by the way, can be treated later.)

Except for the initial injection of Xylocaine, electrodessication is painless—even when the Xylocaine wears off.

TRICHLOROACETIC ACID (TCA) AND PHENOL

TCA and phenol as face peels were discussed in Chapter Six. Isolated keratoses may also be treated with TCA, with the same technique, discomfort, and results described for the face peel. What strength solution to use depends on how thick the lesion is and how deep it goes. A phenol face peel or dermabrasion may be useful with multiple lesions and when the above treatments cannot prevent the visible signs of ultraviolet light damage from recurring quickly. Phenol or a dermabrasion can correct the problem for a longer period of time, but are not often used.

5-FLUOROURACIL

For severe and widespread keratoses on the face, hands, arms, or V of the neck, we recommend chemical treatment with 5-Fluorouracil. 5-Fluorouracil, or 5-F.U., should not be confused with peeling chemicals such as tri-chloroacetic acid or phenol. What is amazing about 5-F.U. is that it seeks out and destroys damaged cells without affecting normal cells in any way. It destroys damaged cells that may not have been apparent to the physician, that might not have been today's lesions but next week's or next month's. Applied to totally healthy skin, 5-F.U. has very little or no effect at all.

Since 1957, 5-Fluorouracil has been used as chemotherapy for internal malignancies. Those patients, who also were suffering from severely sun-damaged skin, found that, while they were being treated with internal 5-F.U., their solar keratoses cleared up. 5-F.U. left their skin smoother and softer. In 1963, it was introduced in a topically applied form. It was on the market only a short time before physicians realized that the side effects that usually accompanied new drugs were not to be seen with 5-F.U. It became accepted as safe and effective quickly and has become the treatment of choice for people with multiple keratoses. 5-Fluorouracil is a great step forward; it has revolutionized the treatment of this particular type of aging skin.

Although 5-Fluorouracil is used at home, usually twice a day for two to six weeks, it is important to use it only under the supervision of a physician, usually a dermatolo-

gist. He should provide detailed instructions for its use at
the first appointment and see you again in about a week to
monitor your progress and make any necessary changes in
instructions. A word of caution: you will look much worse
before you start looking better. In fact, the worse you look,
the better result you can expect in the long run. This is one
of those strange situations in which a severe reaction is
beneficial. During several weeks of using 5-Fluorouracil,
the skin will get red and scaly. When a sufficient reaction
has occurred, you can stop using the 5-F.U. and replace it
with a healing ointment. The redness resembles a very severe sunburn. As it develops, the skin forms a crust and
scabs. Stinging or burning is common as you reach the end
of the 5-F.U. treatment.

Unless you like the lobster look, you will probably want
to make plans to stay out of the limelight for a few weeks.
The redness is too extensive for makeup to be of any use—
though if you do feel the makeup helps there is no harm
using it. Makeup can be applied fifteen to twenty minutes
after the 5-F.U. cream or lotion. Be sure to remove the
makeup completely before you apply the medicine again.
During this time, you must also avoid the sunlight, which
can intensify the reaction.

We *can* keep the inflammation under control by using a
cortisone cream ten to fifteen minutes after using the 5-
Fluorouracil. The only problem with using cortisone—and
there were a number of questions raised about it when it
first came into use—is that we *want* an inflammation as part
of the treatment. It now appears that, at least for solar
keratoses, the cortisone does not interfere with the 5-
Fluorouracil treatment. It does, however, throw a little con-
fusion into the process, since the physician bases the decision on when to stop using the 5-Fluorouracil on the
intensity of the reaction, and if he is using cortisone to re-
tard the reaction he might be misled into stopping the treat-

ment too early or extending it longer than necessary. The answer is to wait a fixed period, say four weeks, regardless of how the inflammation looks. If, despite the cortisone, a sufficiently intense reaction is visible sooner, the treatment can naturally stop sooner.

Solar damage to the lips, which is sometimes too widespread to make freezing or the other methods described above practical, also responds well to 5-Fluorouracil. Anyone who has come home from the beach with sunburned lips knows that swelling, congestion, and occasional small blisters or laceration can result. Chronic exposure to the sun can also effect changes, which usually show up as diffuse, gray-white scaling more prevalent on the lower lip—not chapped lips but interrupted areas of scaling—that does not go away. You can often feel areas of the lip with your finger that are harder than others. Sores may also occur.

For lips, we generally prefer the lower strength liquid instead of the cream. The lip is essentially a mucous membrane, which means that it not only tends to absorb more of the 5-F.U., but that the reaction is dramatic and often quite uncomfortable. The reaction is the same as on the face—redness, then scaling and crusts, and finally some pain or swelling—but it seems to happen more rapidly on the lips. Because the reaction occurs sooner, treatment can be stopped sooner. As with the skin, cortisone cream can be used on the lips in combination with the 5-Fluorouracil. It has been our experience that after 5-F.U. treatment the lips do not heal as rapidly as other areas of the skin, and healing may be accompanied by a little persistent swelling (*edema*). In time, it will all resolve. The keratoses will be gone and the lips back to normal.

Prospective 5-Fluorouracil patients who have seen other patients in their initial reaction stage tend to get scared off. After the treatment is finished, though, the skin gets smooth. It is still red, but the redness disappears in

several weeks. The end result is smooth skin with no keratoses; other signs of aging such as wrinkling and pigmentation are diminished. In most cases, the skin does look
younger. If a few keratoses remain that were overlooked
during treatment, they can be treated by freezing with dry
ice or liquid nitrogen. Skin cancers, we must emphasize,
will not be cured by 5-Fluorouracil and can be removed at a
later date. The patients who have overcome their apprehen-
sion and completed the treatment are very pleased with the
results.

5-Fluorouracil has no serious side effects. Since only a
very small percentage of the drug is absorbed, systemic tox-
icity is not a problem. Some people react more strongly
than others to the drug and may be red for longer. On the
other hand, some people get little or no reaction, and may
need to apply the cream more often or combine the 5-
Fluorouracil treatment with Vitamin A acid (Retin-A®) to
encourage the inflammation. A very small number of people
are allergic to 5-Fluorouracil.

As with dry-ice cryotherapy, some people are tempted
to try a do-it-yourself approach. Once they have gone
through the treatment and have a feel for how it works,
they treat recurring lesions with a little of the left-over
cream. We have one recommendation for left-over 5-F.U.—
throw it away! If, as the do-it-yourselfers do, you treat the
lesion for a few days, just until it gets a little pink, and
then stop, you run the risk of burying an underlying skin
cancer with the new skin that grows back, If the skin cancer is hidden, it can continue to grow undetected. The earlier you treat a skin cancer, the more chance of a cure you
have and, since the lesion is smaller, the better cosmetic results you can expect. It is always preferable to remove a
very small lesion than to treat a larger one. This discussion
should not be taken to mean that we do not advocate the
treatment of isolated lesions with 5-F.U. All it really means

is that we do not advocate you treat them yourself. In the hands of a physician, it's a perfectly good treatment, because he decides when treatment is finished.

To sum up, 5-Fluorouracil has an extremely high success rate and no long-term side effects. Healing is usually complete within six to eight weeks of beginning treatment. It leaves the skin soft, with normal texture and color, and often a little tighter, which makes fine wrinkles less noticeable. Of all therapeutic/cosmetic procedures available, it is the most economical.

QUESTIONS AND ANSWERS

Q. How long does the 5-Fluorouracil treatment last?

A. There's no standard answer, since the amount of actinic or sun damage varies from person to person—as does their willingness to stay out of the sun and avoid further sun damage. In general, the treatment lasts one to five years. Where recurrences happen quickly, there are alternative treatments.

Q. When should I have 5-F.U. treatment?

A. If you mean what time of year, the best time is the winter, when you can more easily avoid sun exposure. If you mean at what point in your life, you can have the treatment at any age and, if lesions recur in a year or two, you can have it again. It is not a question of if you have it now you can't have it later. There is apparently no limit to the number of treatments one can have.

Q. 5-F.U. sounds wonderful. Aren't there any disadvantages?

A. The main disadvantage is the extensive redness and scab formation that occurs during treatment. Since this is difficult to conceal—especially for those who have jobs that put them in regular contact with the public—cosmetic appearance might be considered a disadvantage.

Q. I don't believe there's a drug that has no side effects. There must be some.

A. When we say there are no side effects, we mean the incidence of side effects is so small as to far outweigh any disadvantages. Naturally, there have been occasional side effects reported, such as increased pigmentation that usually goes away by itself, *telangiectasia,* and the tendency to bury skin cancers. But these reports are a handful of the literally millions who have been treated. We might also include as side effects those we expect to see with the treatment—redness, itching, burning, scab formation, and occasional pain.

Q. Why does my friend have a different percentage 5-F.U. cream than I do?

A. 5-F.U. currently comes as a cream or a lotion in strengths of 1 percent, 2 percent, and 5 percent. Except for the lips, we always use the 5 percent cream. (The lips absorb much more cream and the 1 percent liquid is fine.) We have been very happy with 5 percent and see no reason to use the others. Other physicians feel they can get just as good results with a lower percentage. Since the treatment gets worse before it gets better, we can easily monitor its progress and make adjustments as we go along. If you're using a 2 percent concentration and not responding as fast as you should, we could switch you to a 5 percent. We think it's simpler to just start with the 5 percent.

Q. If sunlight intensifies the reaction to 5-FU, and we want a strong reaction, wouldn't it be good to go out in the sun?

A. To intensify the reaction in a person who is progressing normally just means that the treatment would be over sooner. Since we want to use it the full four weeks, to make sure the reaction is complete, sunlight is not usually a good idea. The only exception would be in a person who is not reacting even with increased applications of the medicine. In that case, a little sunshine may help—but in small doses.

Q. I only have a few actinic keratoses and it seems kind of silly to freeze them when only 20 to 25 percent are going to turn into cancer and I can hide them with makeup. Can you tell me why I should bother treating them?

A. Sometimes it's more expensive not to treat something than to treat it. It's more expensive to go into surgery, cut out a cancer, and sew it up later, than to freeze it now for four to ten seconds. The expense is measured not only in dollars but in convenience.

Q. I'm going to have you treat these keratoses on my face, but nobody can see the ones on my legs. Can't I skip them?

A. Since 20 to 25 percent of these keratoses will turn into cancer, the problem is not just cosmetic. We do recommend treatment.

Q. Are there situations where a dermabrasion would be better for keratoses than 5-F.U.?

A. It would seem that 5-F.U. has eliminated the need for dermabrasions in managing multiple recurrent actinic keratoses. But there are some people who get a massive recurrence of keratoses within two or three months of 5-F.U. treatment, though this is very rare. If this is the case, and you are also looking for a dramatic cosmetic improvement of wrinkling and overall facial texture, deep chemical peeling or a dermabrasion would be the answer.

EIGHT

Dermabrasion

If we define surgery as a procedure involving a scalpel —sometimes referred to affectionately as "cold steel"— we can include the dermabrasion in our discussion of alternatives. A dermabrasion is performed with a piece of equipment called a dermabrader or planer. It looks like a dentist's drill with attached brushes, cylinders, serrated wheels, fraises, or burrs for the purpose of sanding off top layers of the skin.

Dermabrasion has had its ups and downs. It was very popular in the mid-fifties for treating acne scars. Then it fell out of favor. Now it is back, still overwhelmingly for acne scars but also for the cosmetic problems of aging skin such as wrinkles and sun spots *(lentigines)*. It can be used on almost any part of the body, though different areas heal at different rates. It can be used to treat sun-damaged skin. And it can be used to treat wrinkles such as frown lines, naso-labial lines, smile lines, vertical wrinkles, and "purse string" wrinkles around the mouth.

After reading about 5-Fluorouracil for the treatment of sun-damaged skin, one might wonder why anyone would undergo the more dramatic procedure of a dermabrasion, which also involves more expense and initial disfigurement. Some people feel the dermabrasion is more effective because it destroys deeper layers of tissue. When it heals, new collagen forms underneath the skin and, since a dermabrasion involves the whole face, the collagen is of a uniform consistency over the whole face. After a dermabrasion, there is less recurrence of solar keratoses than with 5-Fluorouracil, provided the patient is diligent about staying out of the sun or using sunscreens at all times. Some patients get their keratoses back almost immediately after using 5-Fluorouracil. For them, dermabrasion might be an alternative to consider. For those also concerned about their wrinkles, the temporary swelling effect of the dermabrasion does make the wrinkles less noticeable during the healing process and results in long-term improvement as well.

But for treating chronically sun-damaged skin, our personal feeling is that 5-Fluorouracil will replace dermabrasions in most cases for a number of reasons: (1) cost; (2) convenience; (3) fewer and fewer dermatologists are performing dermabrasions and it is a procedure that requires great expertise; and (4) the possibility of complications is much greater with dermabrasion than with 5-Fluorouracil. Nevertheless, there are physicians who will continue to do dermabrasions and do them quite well.

TREATMENT

We start by painting the skin with a purple stain that shows us, first, what area to plane and, second, when we have planed deep enough. Since the stain fills in any pits or marks in the skin, we know whether we have reached the level of the pit or not. The physician works with an assistant. The two make an experienced and interdependent team. The assistant first freezes one area by spraying it from about eighteen inches away with freon, which is not a general anesthetic and is not flammable. When the skin turns white and firm to the touch, the physician goes over the frozen part quickly with the planer and its rapidly spinning brush to remove that layer of skin. They then move on to the next area, working in tandem to complete the entire area in as little as fifteen or twenty minutes (if the team has been working together for some time).

We would expect this kind of procedure to cause quite a bit of pain, but patients report that the pain is minimal and not too bothersome. As the skin thaws, blood begins to ooze out of the capillaries, but it stops quickly, starts to form scabs and superficial crusting, and is not a major problem. Oozing of clear and blood-stained serum may continue even though major hemorrhage of any type rapidly subsides. A thin layer of anesthetic, such as Xylocaine® cream, alleviates a burning sensation. The area is then bandaged.

Oozing may continue for one to two days, and is replaced by crusting when it stops. The crusts consist of the violet serum, blood, and skin cells. Combined with a marked swelling, it makes for an appearance that is, to be frank, shocking. In fact, it is the appearance much more than any pain that will usually incapacitate a patient for ten to fifteen days following the dermabrasion. The crusts start to loosen in seven to ten days and should be allowed to fall off naturally rather than being pulled. The crusts reveal the underlying pink skin—swollen. As with chemical peels, the pinkness takes six to twelve weeks to go away. But the patient must avoid any exposure to sunlight for three to six months—also the case with face peels.

Dermabrasion can be combined with face peels for a more complete treatment. After the peel, dermabrasion can touch up those areas not accessible to the peel. To avoid sharp demarcations, the "feathering" technique is used to blur the line between the peeled and abraded areas. For obvious reasons, dermabrasion is not done around delicate areas like the eyelids.

COMPLICATIONS

If the planing goes too deep, scarring is a possibility. As we learned in the chapter on face peels, the skin needs its supporting structures in order to grow back. Too deep an abrasion destroys these structures. Some areas, like the neck and the sides of the chin, are more likely to scar than others. Scarring is treatable and some resolves by itself.

Pigmentary problems are probably the most common side effect of dermabrasion. Aside from the natural differences from individual to individual in the ability to heal, the major factor is the sun. For that reason, it is absolutely essential to avoid excessive sunshine for at least six months following treatment. Hyperpigmentation occurs much more often than hypopigmentation, but hypopigmentation (that is, a decrease in pigmentation) can occur. Hemorrhage and persistent bleeding can also occur, most likely in those predisposed to bleed or lacking certain clotting factors. This is a very rare occurrence.

Infection is possible but uncommon. The danger of a bacterial infection, of course, is that it would increase the depth of destruction and perhaps leave scarring. But, caught and treated early, bacterial infections are quite easy to control. Other types of infections, such as herpes simplex (cold sores and fever blisters) can also delay the healing process and cause scarring. If you have frequent bouts of herpes or have recently had any kind of vaccination, dermabrasion is probably not for you.

Milia, the white, cyst-like pinpoints mentioned in the

chapter on face peels, occur commonly after dermabrasion, usually several weeks after treatment. They go away by themselves but, since they can take months to do that, the physician will sometimes open them with a small needle and drain them. The procedure is quick, easy, relatively painless, and does not result in scarring.

We mentioned that pain does not usually present a problem, but we realize that pain is subjective. There are many analgesics available, of varying strengths, and it's just a matter of finding the best one to use during the healing process. Contrary to current mythology, drinking alcohol does not deaden the pain, but seems to make it worse.

QUESTIONS AND ANSWERS

Q. I've been thinking of having a dermabrasion but I can't take six months off work and I'm worried about my appearance. What is involved after having a dermabrasion?

A. After the dermabrasion, you usually go home and stay in bed for a couple of days. It's best to sleep on three or four pillows, to keep the head raised and help decrease swelling. Bleeding and oozing may continue for one to two days after which crusts form. These fall off in seven to ten days. Now, about work. We suggest having the dermabrasion done on a Thursday. That gives you one week plus two weekends to recover. In most cases, you can go back to work the next Monday, using a light makeup to cover the redness.

Q. Is dermabrasion covered by insurance?

A. Generally speaking, if dermabrasion is being done for purely cosmetic reasons, no. If it's being done for medical reasons, such as the removal of cancerous or precancerous lesions, it may be covered.

Q. How much does dermabrasion cost?

A. It varies from physician to physician and depends on how large an area is being treated and how many visits are required. It is an expensive procedure and probably getting more expensive because fewer physicians are doing it. It takes quite a bit of expertise.

Q. How much improvement can I expect?

A. Only your physician can attempt to estimate the percentage improvement. It depends on a number of factors. What condition is being treated? How fast do you heal? What is your skin type? A physician needs to draw on all his experience with other patients to make such an estimate. And of course, improvement is subjective. It's the old difference between an optimist and a pessimist. One gets a 20 percent improvement and feels as though it were an 80 percent improvement. The other gets an 80 percent improvement and feels as though it were a 20 percent improvement.

NINE

Silicone

The use of silicone to correct soft tissue defects and wrinkles is controversial, to say the least. It works very well on wrinkles, depressed scars, and faces that are disfigured as the result of certain diseases, and almost any one is a good candidate. But we do not recommend it at this time for two reasons: (1) it is not approved by the Food and Drug Administration, and (2) there is something else now available. Collagen can be injected the same way silicone is, with the advantage that it is approved by the FDA and has, so far, almost no side effects. We will devote an entire chapter to collagen, but for the many people who continue to use or to contemplate the use of silicone, a full discussion is in order.

We would not dismiss silicone simply because it lacks FDA approval. Many commonly used and accepted medical treatments lacked such approval when they were first introduced and some still lack it. With or without the FDA's blessing, silicone has been used for many years, is used at present, and will probably continue to be used.

Nor would we dismiss it simply because it is surrounded by horror stories. Many of the reports describing shifting silicone that slides from the cheek down to the jaw or tissue that breaks down and fills with draining sores are, unfortunately, true. But they are for the most part attributable to improper technique and failure to use pure medical grade silicone.

As with many good things, silicone's early notoriety was a case of too much too soon. In the 1940s and early 1950s glowing reports filtered into the United States from Europe and Japan, based on thousands of cases of people who had been treated with silicone. The problem with these early reports lay not in their authenticity, for many people *had* been treated with immediate and impressive results, but in the failure to allow time for adequate follow-up examinations. Some of the bad results, such as treatments involving the secret "Japanese formula," a mixture of silicone and olive oil, were not reported until later.

The excitement about silicone had two results. Well-controlled laboratory and clinical studies began. But, unfortunately and not unpredictably, many physicians did not wait for more information and began injecting silicone at once. Most of the silicone they used at that time was adulterated. Because of prior experience with injecting paraffin and wax into facial tissues to remove wrinkles, the problem of shifting and migration was not unexpected. Assuming that silicone would also shift, some physicians thought that by adding a material to the silicone, which would cause tissue reaction and scarring, the material could be held in place. (This had also occurred when paraffin and wax were used, causing red, raised tumors in the skin—tragic and untreatable.) The adulteration, then, was premeditated and contained anything that might be expected to cause a reaction—fatty acids, irritant oil, even snake oil. These mixtures, no matter what they contained, were referred to as "silicone," and did much to give silicone a bad name. Recent and on-going studies now indicate it was the additives and not the silicone that caused the problems.

At this time there were also reports of large amounts of adulterated silicone being used for breast augmentations. Injecting a large amount all at the same time often resulted in compression of normal tissue and blockage of the normal lymph drainage channels, leading to permanent and excessive swelling, infection, or, as was often the case, ulceration.

Recent experience with pure medical grade silicone, both in laboratory animals and in humans, has been quite different. Investigators now feel that medical grade silicone, if used properly, is both safe and effective. Side effects are rare. There are no statistics on how many physicians are now using medical grade silicone but, from patients we have seen who have had such treatment, we believe its use is widespread. Since medical grade silicone can be stored indefinitely at room temperature and can be repeatedly sterilized without damage to its chemical characteristics, practitioners who obtained large amounts when it was still available in this country have a generous and perfectly functional supply. It can also be purchased in Mexico and other countries.

As the use of silicone is now established and can be expected to continue, we will discuss the right way to use it. Silicone has been around for many years. An English chemist introduced the term, using letters from the chains of silicon (an element), oxygen, and methane (a hydrocarbon) that make up the mixture. Medical grade fluid silicone is odorless, colorless, and clear. It has an oily feel, something like mineral oil in its viscosity (resistance to flow). "Medical grade" refers to the particle purity of a sterile preparation of a known viscosity.

One unquestionably legitimate use for silicone is in treating hemifacial atrophy, a disease process that can start in infancy and leave one half of an otherwise normal face disfigured by a marked lack of underlying tissue and large indented areas. Silicone has been very effective in filling out the indentations. On a less drastic scale, it has been effective in filling out wrinkles and scars, especially indented scars such as those resulting from acne.

In this book, we are primarily interested in its cosmetic use. As with any cosmetic procedure, it is important to know before you commit yourself what the side effects are and what results you can realistically expect.

Silicone is injected with a hypodermic needle. The pain is no worse than any normal injection; the silicone itself does not cause any pain. There is always the possibility that, since it is impossible to see beneath the skin, the physician might puncture a blood vessel while making the injection. This can lead to discomfort from local bleeding, leakage of blood under the skin, a little redness, and a slight swelling. Of course, some swelling is the whole point of the procedure—that's how the underlying tissue is raised. But there are two types of swelling, that is, the intended swelling and the temporary swelling that would accompany any kind of injection.

Sedation is usually not necessary. Before injection, the area to be treated is well cleaned to remove germs and debris from the skin. To place the silicone, there are two techniques, depending on what kind of problem is being corrected. The serial or multiple puncture technique uses a very fine needle (the smaller the needle, of course, the less pain) to make a series of injections along the problem line. In the case of a wrinkle or smile line between the lip and the nose, for example, the physician would simply follow the line of the wrinkle, making small injections and depositing small amounts of silicone to raise the entire wrinkle. The fanning technique uses one injection with the needle running parallel to the skin's surface. As it is slowly withdrawn the physician can control the distribution of the silicone. The question is not whether one technique is better than the other, but rather, which is appropriate for the type of problem being treated. The line, size, and shape of the defect will determine which technique is to be used. Anesthesia is usually not used because the presence of anesthetic in the same area would also affect the shape of the skin and thus present problems in determining how much silicone to use and where.

Now, the question you have all been waiting for. How large is the needle? Very, very small—usually 30 gauge, less than an inch long, with a 1 cc syringe with rings for the physician's fingers to facilitate control. For special occasions requiring larger amounts of silicone, a 3 cc syringe may be used. The injection should reach the hypodermal level which, you will recall, is where the dermis meets the subcutaneous fat. The physician can make sure he has not encountered a blood vessel by drawing back on the hypodermic. If the needle has punctured a blood vessel, blood will enter the syringe and it is time to try a different spot.

It is better to inject too little than too much. If more is needed, it can be injected in a second session. Silicone should be injected in small quantities, from as little as 0.01 cc to the more common 0.08 to 0.20 at any one time. (For larger defects such as hemifacial atrophy, where a fanning technique would be used, larger amounts of silicone would be deposited.) Using small amounts greatly decreases the danger of the silicone drifting. If it seems that the physician has not injected enough, it is because a fibro-plastic reaction will later increase the fullness slightly. Correct procedure is to inject slightly less than necessary, wait for the reaction, and add more silicone in a second session if needed. For optimal results, at least five days should pass between injections. In practice, it's usually a week or longer.

After the injection, pressure is applied moderately to

the area to help the skin retain the fluid silicone and to stop the bleeding, if a blood vessel has been damaged, before swelling or discoloration occurs. Some physicians may use an instrument to vibrate the area for up to eight minutes in an effort to disperse the silicone and do away with bumps. There has been some discussion as to whether this is really necessary or not.

When the procedure has been done correctly, with very small amounts of fluid silicone, the area should feel quite natural after the injection. There should be little sensation or sensitivity unless large amounts have been used, in which case there may be a rubbery consistency. No particular care is necessary after the treatment other than common sense. Naturally, you want to avoid any trauma to the area. Avoid facial massages for at least a month after the last injection. Use simple cosmetics or makeup.

There are a few possible adverse reactions to silicone injection. Everybody has a different tolerance for the pain of a needle and, although the smallest gauge needles are used to keep the pain to a minimum, pain may occur in some individuals. The injection by needle may cause a slight swelling, but this should go away after a day or two. And there is, as we mentioned, the possibility of hitting a blood vessel. Blood that leaks under the skin may turn a dark color, the classic example being a black eye. On occasion, there may be some redness at the site of the injection, due to irritation, but it is usually gone after a couple of hours and can be covered easily with makeup. An injection too close to the surface can also cause redness, and this kind may persist. It can be treated with anti-inflammatory creams. In rare cases, pigmentation changes may give the skin a bluish tint or even a brownish-yellow pigmentation. This is due to injecting the silicone too close to the surface and is temporary.

Over-correction, over-injection, and not waiting long

enough between injections can cause problems. Injections too close to the surface can also cause what we call a *peau d'orange* stippling. A goosebump effect like the peel of an orange, *peau d'orange* was very common in the early days of using silicone for breast augmentation. If the silicone does not disperse adequately, it can leave beading or nodulation that can persist for a long time. If it does not go away by itself, a local injection of cortisone, an anti-inflammatory medicine, is indicated. Excessive elevation or over-correction may also respond to cortisone.

The problem of embolism is a little more serious. An embolism occurs when a substance injected into a blood vessel travels along the blood vessel, becomes lodged at some point in the blood vessel, and cuts off blood to that area of the skin or body. If the physician uses small amounts of silicone with frequent checks, as we suggested above, to make sure he is not in a blood vessel before he injects the silicone, there should be no problem. If an embolism does occur, it could be felt as a headache, as local pain, or as pain at a site far away from the injection. When silicone was being injected in large amounts (literally hundreds of milliliters) for breast augmentations, embolism to organ systems and, in some cases, fatalities occurred.

There are a few cases in which silicone should definitely not be used. It is now felt that silicone should not, under any circumstances, be *injected* into the breast. The current acceptable practice is to use silicone in plastic bags, entirely enclosed, and implant the entire bag into the breast. In addition to the problems already mentioned if loose silicone is injected into the breast, it can interfere with the detection of possibly cancerous masses later. We might mention at this point that there has never been any indication that silicone itself is carcinogenic. It has been used for years in the body—as part of synthetic heart valves, to mention one example—without complications.

Silicone should not be used on the eyelids, where the skin is too thin, or for certain types of scars. Some scars respond well to silicone; some do not, and the judgment is best left to a skilled practitioner. But we might mention that the small, deep acne scars often referred to as icepick scars usually cannot be raised with silicone. They are called icepick scars because they look like they were made with an icepick that was stuck into the skin and left a hole. The scar is usually so embedded that it cannot be raised by injecting silicone underneath. If silicone is injected, it will only succeed in raising the level of the entire scar, so that it looks the same as it did before, except that it has a small bump underneath.

Silicone can be used in combination with dermabrasions, chemical peels, and facelifts, but it should be remembered that injection of fluid silicone or any other substance is not a substitute for plastic surgery. It cannot create new structures. It cannot correct laxity or sagging of tissues. It is at best a means of improving some long-standing defects or making wrinkles and other soft tissue defects less noticeable.

Even after many years of use, silicone is still considered an investigational drug. The fact that it is still investigational means that there is more to learn about it, even though it does appear that, when used correctly, it is safe.

QUESTIONS AND ANSWERS

Q. How do you find a physician who does silicone injections?

A. We have no doubt that there are many physicians who do silicone injections, but we have seen no advertisements nor do we know of anyone in our area who does it. At one time the Dow Chemical Corporation, the maker of pure medical grade silicone, had set up a joint endeavor with the

Food and Drug Administration involving some twenty-six investigators. Either the FDA or Dow Chemical might be able to refer one of these investigators. Another avenue might be the better beauty salons. For some reason, they seem to know more about what is going on with silicone than physicians do.

Q. How long has silicone been used in humans?

A. It has been used for about thirty years in Japan and almost that long in the United States. Disregarding the early failures due to impure material and improper technique, the American experience over the last fifteen years with silicone has given excellent results.

Q. Are there uses you did not mention in the chapter for silicone?

A. Injectable silicone has been used for fifteen years in a study of augmentation for problems of the diabetic foot. It can give the foot a synthetic cushion as a treatment for corns, calluses, and scar tissue. During these fifteen years, only one or two cases of fluid drift, which was asymptomatic, have been reported, and those were early cases involving too much injection. Complications such as infection, tumor formation, or rejection of the material have not been reported.

Q. If I get silicone injections over a period of time will they dissolve?

A. There is no indication in the research that a living organism can absorb or metabolize silicone fluid.

Q. Can silicone injections cause or result in cancer?

A. In a study of over sixteen thousand breast augmentations, almost all done with silicone, there were no reported neoplasms. Hundreds of thousands of people live with silicone rubber shunts in their heads for treatment of water on the brain. Many patients have synthetic silastic heart valves or bands encircling detached retinas that are made of silicone. So, in solid form, silicone has been used in thousands of patients for a long time without evidence of carcinogenesis.

Q. You say silicone cannot be broken down by organisms, but I've heard it does disappear with time. Is this true?

A. We don't really know what happens to silicone in the long run. Clinical observation has shown that the amount of silicone can decrease gradually and finally disappear from the tissues, necessitating another injection.

Q. Do you recommend silicone injections for the correction of my wrinkles?

A. This is a difficult question to answer. First of all, you must decide for yourself if you want your wrinkles corrected. In the last analysis, cosmetic surgery involves a personal evaluation. How much do you want to change the way you look and what are you willing to go through to change? We have never used silicone in our office, but we have seen excellent results with it. We have also followed the literature closely, so we know about the bad results, too. If you are considering silicone injections, you must find someone whose experience and technique you can trust.

TEN

Collagen

Of all the recent developments in cosmetic dermatology, the advent of the Zyderm™ Collagen Implant is easily the most exciting. A safe, simple, and effective way to eliminate unsightly scars, and wrinkles—be they the result of acne, surgery, trauma, or aging—has been, until now, nothing more than a dream. Many techniques have been tried in an effort to eliminate imperfections and smooth the contour of the skin, including injection of various materials to fill out lines and wrinkles and elevate depressed areas of the skin, but they have not been entirely satisfactory.

The Zyderm™ Collagen Implant—not to be confused with cosmetics containing collagen for application to the surface of the skin—is a substance similar to the skin's own collagen. It can be injected directly into the skin, at the precise location and depth necessary for best cosmetic results, and, once injected, becomes part of the skin's natural support structure. Since it is made from collagen taken from cows it must be specially processed, so it does not trigger the body's immune defense system, as many foreign substances do. Reaction to foreign substances has been the main problem with previous implants; even if the body did not reject them entirely, they could become isolated or enclosed by the surrounding tissue and, in many cases, migrate from the location where they were originally injected to other parts of the skin. So what is the ideal implant? The ideal implant is a substance resembling the body's own structural protein, collagen, something the body can recognize as its own. Once new cells and blood vessels grow into the implant and make it an organic part of the skin, the body can be persuaded to accept the implant as part of its own support network. Zyderm™ Collagen Implant comes very close to fitting this description. It has enabled us to fill in and correct many imperfections that could previously be treated only with silicone.

Before examining the Zyderm™ Collagen Implant, we should first understand the function of the skin's own collagen. Collagen is the protein found most abundantly in the skin's connective tissue. Its primary function is to hold the body tissues together; in fact, "collagen" comes from the Greek word for glue. This "glue," tough and pliant, is found in skin, cartilage, tendons, muscles, ligaments, artery walls, nerve sheets, bone, and most internal organs. It accounts for almost a third of the human body's protein and might be called the body's number one building block or "nature's nylon."

Collagen is no stranger to the medical laboratory. It is used in surgical "cat-gut" sutures and hemostatic agents, both designed to break down and disappear in the body, and in heart valves and contraceptive sponges, which are designed to stay intact. In a less pure form, collagen shows up in edible sausage casings, gelatin, and, of course, topical collagen face creams.

In the skin, collagen fibers make up about 90 percent of

the dermis, interweaving like threads in a cloth to form an intricate lattice-work support structure for the surrounding tissues. Cells and blood vessels from the tissue grow into and mingle with the injected collagen which acts as a support structure. Collagen fiber is responsible for giving the skin its texture and contour. In young, healthy skin, the collagen allows enough stretching to be practical but not enough to be unattractive. Acne, chicken pox, infection, and surgical incision can damage the collagen structure, leaving scars, pits, and wrinkles.

The Zyderm™ Collagen Implant, viewed through a microscope, closely resembles the structure of interwoven fibers normally found in healthy skin—including the cells and blood vessels from neighboring tissue that grow into the implant and make it a viable part of the skin. The implant behaves like normal, healthy connective tissue—that is, like normal, healthy skin. Because it becomes an integrated part of the growing skin, the implant does not migrate to other areas.

While injectable collagen can be used to correct a variety of soft-tissue defects, readers of this book will be most interested in its use with wrinkles. Of course, those who hoped their wrinkles were barely noticeable may be upset to learn that not only have physicians noticed the wrinkles, they have given them names. Those wrinkles that appear on the forehead between the eyes are known as "glabellar lines." Wrinkles running from the nose downward towards the side of the face—grin lines—are known as the "nasal labial fold." Glabellar lines and the nasal labial fold seem to respond the best to collagen implants. In fact, one can expect a 70 to 80 percent improvement in those areas, which is all anyone would want since a 100 percent improvement would look quite unnatural. Tiny creases in the surface of the skin or wrinkles due to an excess of skin do not respond well to collagen implants. The horizontal lines on the forehead will respond. We do not treat folds along the neck. The fine-line wrinkles around the mouth, often referred to as "purse-string" wrinkles, are somewhat more difficult to correct, but can definitely be improved. Because the skin is thinner around the eyelids, collagen implants require extreme caution there.

How long the results last depends, of course, on the individual and on what kind of problem has been treated. A collagen implant can reverse the visible effects of aging but it cannot reverse aging itself. Because it is a natural skin-like substance, it ages like skin. Disease and muscle activity, like frowning or pursing the lips, will continue to break down the skin. Thus, to maintain any correction, periodic supplemental injections are necessary. Clinical tests of Zyderm™ Collagen, in which we participated, showed that 30 percent of patients undergoing implants showed no change after eighteen months. About 20 percent needed minor supplemental implants after six to twenty-four months; these patients lost about 10 to 20 percent of their correction every six months. From these figures, it is fair to say that, especially if the problem treated is due to an on-going process like aging, supplemental injections would be required between six and twenty-four months after the initial treatment course.

Collagen injections do not replace facelifts, dermabrasions, or chemical peels. Collagen has no effect on sagging skin. It can, however, be used in conjunction with other procedures, to fine-tune the result. The Collagen Corporation recommends a three- to six-month wait between collagen implants and dermabrasions or chemical peels. Which to do first is a hard question to answer. If you have severe wrinkling, it makes sense to have the peel first, see how effective it is, and then see what areas could benefit from injecting collagen. On the other hand, some patients who did not have severe wrinkling and underwent collagen implants first found the results so appealing that a chemical peel was not necessary after all. The physician who will perform the procedure is the best source of advice in making the decision.

We are often asked how we can inject cow collagen into humans without triggering the body's rejection mechanism. As the public becomes more knowledgeable about the dazzling organ transplants produced by modern medicine, it has also learned about the body's foreign tissue rejection mechanism. The collagen molecule is quite similar in all mammals, and the purifying and processing that bovine (cow) collagen undergoes, before becoming Zyderm™ Collagen Implant, increases the similarities. Technically speaking, the difference between a molecule of cow collagen and a molecule of human collagen is a large globular area at the end of the fibers known as a telopeptide. The processing removes the telopeptides. To put it another way, the collagen molecule is composed of a helix—strands wrapping around each other—with a telopeptide tail at the top and bottom. During the Zyderm™ Collagen processing, these strands are unwrapped. Since the telopeptide is primarily responsible for the differences between collagen in different animals, removing it removes the essential ingredient that labels it cow collagen as opposed to human collagen and makes it acceptable for implanting in humans.

TREATMENT

Vascular grafts and heart valves, derived from cow and pig collagen, have been surgically implanted in the human body for many years with good results. Injectible collagen has eliminated the need for surgical implantation because it comes suspended in what we call a dispersion, a gel-like solution of salt water. This dispersion can be injected directly into the skin with a very small needle. No surgery or incision is necessary.

In the syringe, the collagen is milky white, odorless, and the consistency of soft paste. It is injected directly into scarred or wrinkled areas of the face and, when the dispersion warms to body temperature, it condenses. The collagen fibers reconstitute to their helical strand to become a natural part of the skin.

The first step in treatment is a consultation with the physician—usually a dermatologist, plastic surgeon, or ear-nose-and-throat specialist. The physician will take a detailed medical history, looking for any conditions that would rule you out for the procedure. Rheumatoid arthritis, lupus erythematosis, dermatomyositis, polymyositis, and other autoimmune diseases in you or any member of your immediate family make you more likely than most to develop a reaction to the collagen implant and make treatment in your case unwise. The collagen dispersion contains a small amount of lidocaine, an anesthetic, so if you are allergic to lidocaine, you would not be a good candidate for implantation. It is not yet known whether Zyderm™ reacts with substances, like silicone, that may have been injected into the skin on previous occasions. For that reason, it is not advised at present that former silicone recipients undergo a collagen implantation. This may change, though, as a result of research now in progress. Injectable collagen is *not* used for breast augmentation or for implantation in bones, tendons, ligaments, or muscles.

The second step in treatment is a skin test to determine whether you are sensitive to the collagen implant material. After an injection of a small amount (0.1 cc) of the collagen into your forearm, you will be asked to keep a careful eye on the area for four weeks, looking for signs of allergic reaction. Redness and swelling a few hours after the injection is to be expected—but if the redness and swelling persist or if you notice any unusual itching or hardness around the test area at any time during the four-week test period, you must tell your physician.

Less than 3 percent of all patients fail to pass this skin test. If you show no signs of sensitivity after four weeks, you are ready for treatment, which can be done in the doctor's office. It starts with the patient sitting in an upright position under a bright light; wrinkles are less noticeable when we lie down. With the light revealing the skin in all its glory, or lack of, the physician uses a colored marking pen to outline the areas he will later inject.

The injection involves a little discomfort, though the presence of the anesthetic lidocaine in the dispersion helps numb the area temporarily. Before the numbing takes effect, the lidocaine will sting a bit. We have treated many patients and no one yet has asked to have the treatment stopped because of discomfort.

Since the collagen dispersion is 70 percent salt water, which will be absorbed later, the physician tries to inject as much of the substance as possible. At first it will look like over-correction, but after the water is absorbed, the volume of the collagen remaining in place is only 25 to 30 percent of the volume of the dispersion originally injected. The physician follows his marking-pen outline with the needle, making multiple injections along the line of the wrinkle or other defect. The more he can inject, swelling the tissue to its maximum, the more successful the first treatment will be, and the less need there will be for follow-up treatments. There are no cases on record of over-correction that stays in place permanently, though in areas where the skin is very thin, such as the areas around the eyes or lips, the over-correction will disappear at a slower rate. For that reason, these areas should be treated very conservatively—if they are to be treated at all—and should not be over-corrected.

Collagen can be safely implanted in the connective tissues at any depth, but it is most effective close to the surface, high in the dermis. When the area near the surface is over-corrected, the result is often a stippled, goose-bump effect we call *peau d'orange* or orange peel coupled with a whiteness of the tissue. Both phenomena should disappear within hours after the treatment, and the swelling, rather than being cause for alarm, should be taken as a sign of the physician's success in implanting a significant amount of collagen in the skin. Injecting collagen is something like blowing up a balloon. You deliberately overinflate the balloon because you know you will lose some of the air when you tie the nozzle. The physician deliberately over-corrects or overinjects the skin with collagen knowing that, as the water is absorbed, some of the volume will be lost.

Unlike surgical procedures, collagen implantation involves a short recovery period and very little time lost from work or in hiding. The skin suffers a minimum of trauma and disruption. Don't be surprised if, after the first treatment, you see no noticeable correction. Often the function of the first treatment is not so much to fill out the tissues as to stretch them and soften them so that the second treatment will be much easier. It's a little like ironing a shirt. On the first pass you may smooth out the shirt but you can still see wrinkles. As you continue ironing, the wrinkles disappear. Most people begin to see very good results by their second or third treatment. Improvement seems to occur all of a sudden. It is not uncommon for a patient to be less than excited after treatment number two or three only to be ecstatic about the results after treatment number four. At the end of one such treatment for acne scarring, we said to the happy patient, "We have filled all the acne scars we're going to treat today. We still have some collagen left. Should we start treating some wrinkles?" She replied, "No, I want to get rid of my adolescence before we tackle the sunrise of my middle age."

RESULTS

The Zyderm™ Collagen Implant has been extensively tested in both animal and human studies over the past seven years. We participated, with seven hundred other dermatologists and plastic surgeons, in clinical tests from September 1979 to July 1981, involving some nine thousand patients. Careful records were kept and analyzed for five thousand of the patients, leading to approval by the Food and Drug Administration in July 1981. We would like to thank Susan Kweskin of the Collagen Corporation for making available to us the data and analysis made during that time.

Of those cases in which collagen was implanted to treat aging skin, 48 percent involved furrows and wrinkles like glabellar frown lines and nasal labial folds. After the first treatment, they reported "good" correction, which they defined as 40 to 60 percent, and after three treatments, they reported "very good" correction. "Very good" correction required between 2 and 5 cc of Zyderm™ implant.

Of course, everyone is different. Statistics can serve only as a general guideline. How many visits you will need and how much correction you can expect depends on a number of factors: how deep your wrinkles are, how much underlying skin damage exists, and how much collagen is used, to name a few. Similarly, how long the correction can be expected to last is an individual matter, influenced by factors such as what technique is used, how much over-correction is achieved (the more the area is over-corrected at the time of implantation, the fewer implantations will be required), and how elastic the tissue is in the area being corrected. Attempts to build up tissue beyond its normal limits—for example, using collagen to augment the chin—are not usually successful, since they put too much stress on the implant. But a scar area that may not seem treatable at first may subsequently respond well. An initial injection of small amounts of collagen often results in softening of the tissue and makes it more receptive to later injections of collagen.

SAFETY

Although Zyderm™ Collagen Implant is very new, extensive tests have shown it to be extremely safe. Safety has not been established for pregnant women, children, or infants, and we have no information on long-term effects beyond the three years it has been used on humans. Nevertheless, the information we do have from the Collagen Corporation is impressive.

Only 3 percent of patients involved in the study had adverse reactions to the pretreatment skin test, usually involving the expected redness, swelling, tenderness, or hardness. Of these, only a very small percentage developed systemic complaints (arthralgia, itching, rashes, or swelling), and all responded to treatment.

Of patients who received Zyderm™ Collagen Implants, very few developed responses associated with treatment. Temporary painless bruising involving the small vessels around the site of the injection occasionally occurs after injection of any kind of material that distends the tissue. Temporary or recurring hardness and swelling, when it occasionally occurred, lasted only a few hours and is often associated with drinking alcohol, prolonged exposure to the sun or to heat, and flare-ups of hay fever. These reactions clear up by themselves and do not interfere with the effect of the collagen treatment.

Half of the adverse reactions occurred in patients who had had a positive reaction to the skin test that went unreported and resulted in swelling, redness, hardness, and/or hives in the area of the implant. The other reactions included infection, redness, swelling, and cold sores in areas of previous cold sores. We have the screening procedure of the skin test to thank for the very low figure of 1.3 percent adverse reactions to the actual treatment. Given the importance of the skin test, we emphasize that, even though 50 percent of all test reactions occur in the first 24 hours and over 70 percent occur in the first 72 hours, the test site should be watched for a full four weeks, as recommended, before proceeding with treatment. Approximately 0.6% of patients became sensitive to Zyderm™ Collagen Implant during the first four treatments.

None of the reported adverse responses has been dangerous. Many of the reactions lasted only two to three weeks, though some persisted for three to four months, and one persisted eight months. These reactions were primarily cosmetic problems, which did cause distress and frustration for the patients, but did not threaten their general health. All resolved in time with no dangerous results.

COST

In our office, we figure the cost of a treatment at our time plus the cost of the material to us. At the time of this writing there is, to our knowledge, only one company that manufactures the material, and it is located in Palo Alto, California. Since the collagen must be kept cold during storage, costs of transportation are high, and they get higher the farther away from Palo Alto one lives. As these costs go up, our costs go up. We cannot speak for other physicians and we know that they have different ways of calculating their costs. We would suggest calling the offices of several physicians and simply asking them directly what they charge. Some sample questions: How much is the skin test? How much for ½ cc and how much for 1 cc? Does the cost include an office visit or is that extra? Don't bother to ask over the phone how many cc's you will need. Obviously, that requires a visual examination by an experienced physician after the initial treatment.

Some people are never satisfied. We have seen patients we thought had only fair results from a dermabrasion rave about it. We have seen great results shrugged off as barely acceptable. All we can say is that, of all the patients we have treated who have had an adequate number of treatments, we have had no complaints. The best way to keep a patient pleased is to keep the expectations realistic.

QUESTIONS AND ANSWERS

Q. I've never had problems, but some close relatives have histories of asthma, hay fever, and skin disease. Does this mean I can't have collagen treatment?

A. Asthma, hay fever, and skin disease are classically seen with a phenomenon called atopic diathesis. It does not mean you can't have treatment, but it does mean you should be very critical of the skin test. If there's even a hint of a reaction that's questionable, it should be repeated in the other arm. People with this kind of history have an increased incidence of allergic hypersensitivity.

Q. After I had my skin test, I found out a blood relative has rheumatoid arthritis. What should I do?

A. Be sure to tell your physician so he does not begin treatment. As for the test area, it is so small that adverse problems are unlikely.

Q. What would be considered an untoward test reaction?

A. Any change in the original test injection site such as increased redness, hardness, tenderness, or swelling, with or without accompanying itching, that persists for more than six hours or that appears more than twenty-four hours following implantation and/or the onset of rash, joint pains, or muscle pains.

Q. Is discoloration one of the side effects of Zyderm™ Collagen Implant?

A. Yes. We see two types. One is the blanching that occurs as a result of the treatment and lasts five to ten minutes at most. The other is bruising as a result of the needle breaking a blood vessel. Leakage of blood in the second case causes a purplish discoloration that lasts a little longer but is not permanent.

Q. Is there any type of skin that makes the treatment less effective or more difficult to administer?

A. People with very large pores may find that, when the medicine is injected, it leaks out through a pore and does not stay in the skin. This doesn't mean you can't be treated, but it does mean that you may need to have more injections until the physician can find some place to inject without having the collagen come out of a pore.

Q. Once I start treatment, how often can I be treated?

A. The same area should not be treated more than once every two weeks. If you're treating different areas, you can be treated as often as you like. It's no problem to wait longer.

Q. Is there a maximum amount of collagen one can have?

A. The Collagen Corporation feels at this time that the total volume of implanted collagen should not exceed 30 cc in any given patient over a twelve-month period.

Q. I've had collagen implants around the eye and it still feels lumpy even though it's been a couple of weeks. Why is this?

A. There has never been a reported case of over-correction with a collagen implant, because of its high water content. In certain areas, there is minimal tissue stress. The very soft, extensible skin around the eyes is a good example. The collagen implant can sit there for some time without any pressure. You may help it along by supplying slight pressure or just wait for it to resolve with time.

Q. I like my collagen implant and want to really finish things off with a chemical peel. How long do I have to wait?

A. The Collagen Corporation recommends that there be a three to six month lapse between the collagen implant and the chemical peel.

Q. At this time, are there any legal restrictions on who can administer Zyderm™ Collagen Implants?

A. Federal regulations restrict the sale, distribution, or use of collagen to physicians who are board-certified in their specialty, have participated in a Collagen Corporation training program, and have advanced training in soft tissue anatomy and physiology and/or training and experience in alternative methods of soft tissue contour restoration. As a result of an article in a national publication in which we were quoted, we received letters from people all over the country asking where they could get collagen treatment. Our answer was either to call local dermatologists, plastic surgeons, and medical associations, or to write the Collagen Corporation at 2455 Faber Place, Palo Alto, CA 94303.

JAMES H. STERNBERG, M.D.
A MEDICAL CORPORATION
THOMAS H. STERNBERG, M.D.
10921 WILSHIRE BOULEVARD, SUITE 410
LOS ANGELES, CALIFORNIA 90024
208-8688

DERMATOLOGY   November 24, 1981

<u>Collagen Questionnaire</u>
Warnings, Precautions, and Restrictions

1)   Are you now pregnant or are you planning to get pregnant during the treatment program?   Yes_____   No_____

2)   The implantation of Zyderm carries an inherent, yet minimal, risk of infection, as does any procedure involving injections into the skin. I am willing to accept this risk.   Yes_____   No_____

3)   Because significant data have not been gathered beyond 3 years of clinical experience, the safety of this product beyond this time period is not known. I understand the above (#3) statement and wish to proceed with the treatment.   Yes_____   No_____

4)   Do you personally or any of your immediate family (blood relatives) have a history of: (the doctor will explain each disease)

A)	Rheumatoid Arthritis	Yes_____	No_____
B)	Psoriatic Arthritis	Yes_____	No_____
C)	Lupus Erythematosus (discoid or systemic)	Yes_____	No_____
D)	Dermatomyositis	Yes_____	No_____
E)	Polymyositis	Yes_____	No_____
F)	Hashimoto's Thyroiditis	Yes_____	No_____
G)	Graves' Disease	Yes_____	No_____
H)	Polyarteritis Nodusa	Yes_____	No_____
I)	Progressive systemic Sclerosis (Scleroderma)	Yes_____	No_____
J)	Ulcerative Colitis	Yes_____	No_____
K)	Crohn's Disease	Yes_____	No_____
L)	Sjogren's Syndrome	Yes_____	No_____
M)	Reiter's Syndrome	Yes_____	No_____
N)	Mixed Connective Tissue Disease	Yes_____	No_____

6)   Do you have a lidocaine (Xylocaine) hypersensitivity?

                                        Yes_____   No_____

7)   Do you have a history of Anaphalactoid Reactions?

                                        Yes_____   No_____

8)   Have you had previous treatment with other injectible materials e.g.
silicone, paraffin, etc.?   Yes_____   No_____

I have completely understood all the above questions before answering them and wish to commence treatment with Zyderm™ Collagen Implant.

                                        Signed _____

Witness   Date _____
_____

ELEVEN

Pigmentary Changes, Blood Vessels, Cancer, and Other Woes

The office procedures we have described in this book are useful in treating many of the miscellaneous problems that occur as the skin ages. In this chapter we examine problems associated with blood vessels (primarily dilation and easy bruisability), pigmentary changes (including freckles and liver spots)—and skin cancer.

TELANGIECTASIA

With sun damage, blood vessels lose the ability to contract. When they become permanently dilated, they may form a network of fine superficial lines that, when we were less careful of our vocabulary, was known as "senile telangiectasia" and now is called simply telangiectasia. It usually occurs on the cheeks, and from a distance can pass itself off as a healthy, rosy glow. On closer inspection, though, the blood vessels become quite obvious, especially on those long-suffering people with fair skin and hair.

The best treatment for telangiectasia is with an electric needle. We call it an electrosurgical tip. It is very similar to the needle or wire used in electrolysis. Attached to the electrodessicator, with the power at its lowest setting, the needle touches the blood vessel, giving an instantaneous sensation of a mild shock. The electric current causes the blood vessel to coagulate and disappear from view. Since local anesthesia can cause the blood vessels to temporarily disappear, we must perform the procedure without anesthesia in order to be able to locate the blood vessels we want to treat.

In treating an isolated lesion, the results are immediately apparent. If we could offer immediate results for acne or wrinkles, we would be preparing our Nobel Prize acceptance speeches right now; this treatment is one of the few in all dermatology that works so well. Not that there are not problems: a certain percentage of the blood vessels will reopen and thus reappear and require another treatment. There is a slight possibility of leaving a pitted scar at the site of treatment—but this side effect is quite rare, especially on the cheeks. It is more likely to occur, if it occurs at all, in treating spider telangiectasia, which are usually larger and may require slightly more electricity.

Cutaneous telangiectasia of the lower legs, a common complaint in our office, usually consists of dilated blood vessels, which are too large to respond to the electrosurgical tip. The blood vessels usually form purplish linear groups, often near deeper varicose veins—especially at the point these vessels meet, where pressure may be greater. They sometimes form a starburst pattern and can occur anywhere on the leg, including the ankles and feet. Blame it on your genes in most cases, though it can be associated with trauma in people who work standing up for long periods of time. This form of telangiectasia presents no danger, though it is at times unsightly.

Injection of a salt water solution directly into the blood

vessels has worked well as a treatment for many years. Not all physicians perform the procedure, so check with the dermatologist or cardiovascular surgeon before making an appointment. Simply put, the salt water solution causes the cells that make up the blood vessels to dry out and die. Some time after the injection, sometimes as long as a month to three months, the blood vessels close. The injection itself may cause either a slight stinging or a feeling of warmth. Pressure dressings may need to be applied afterward and kept on until bedtime. Prolonged standing or physical exertion should be avoided during the first twenty-four to forty-eight hours after the injection. It should be kept in mind that, naturally, the injection gets rid of existing blood vessels but has no effect on the formation of more.

Side effects may include a slight blistering at the site of injection caused by leakage of the saline solution out of the blood vessel and into the surrounding skin. It should heal rapidly but occasionally leaves some residual pigmentation. If bruising occurs, it can last a month or two but will heal completely. On rare occasions, a clot forms at the site of the injection. It is not dangerous and heals quickly after the clot is removed.

ANGIOMAS

Cherry, ruby, or senile (who said that?) angiomas are three names for the same thing, usually visible as bright red, dome-shaped papules as small as pinpoints. They have no other symptoms; that is, if you couldn't see them you would never know they were there. They have no malignant potential and are not otherwise dangerous. Once they start to appear, usually on the upper trunk, they will continue to appear. If, for cosmetic reasons, one wishes to have them removed, very small ones respond well to the epilating needle used for telangiectasia. Larger ones may require electrodessication and curettage, discussed in Chapter Seven.

PURPURA

As sun damage wreaks its havoc with the skin's connective tissues, the blood vessels lose their supporting structure and become more susceptible to bruising. Blood leakage under the skin is responsible for the bruise, which we call purpura. Since sun damage is the first link in the purpura chain, it stands to reason that purpura is most common on the hands and arms, which are most exposed not only to the sun but to the bumps and minor collisions with the rest of the world. "*I* never bump my arms," is a refrain we hear constantly in our office, usually from women patients with badly bruised arms who then proceed to hook their purses over their arms and march out the door with the purse straps slapping away at the arms—exactly where the bruises are.

Vitamin C and zinc are sometimes recommended for treatment of purpura by the theory that a Vitamin C deficiency can enhance bruisability and that zinc often helps wounds heal. Neither has ever worked on our patients. The best treatment we can recommend is to avoid the bruises in the first place by wearing long sleeves and exercising caution.

Venous lakes—localized accumulations of widened veins soft to the touch and usually blue in color—have no malignant potential. They occur most commonly in men, usually on the ears but also on the neck, face, and lower lip. They can be removed by electrodessication and curettage if they present a cosmetic problem, but this may leave a circular scar about the size of the original lesion.

LIVER SPOTS (LENTIGINES)

Liver spots are a conspicuous and undeniable sign of aging. If you have a fair complexion and have spent your life soaking up the sun, there is almost no way to avoid them. They first appear at thirty to forty years of age as flat round or oval marks that are light brown or tan and have distinct margins—that is to say, the pigmentation does not blend into the surrounding tissue. They have no texture or feel. In fact, if you were to close your eyes and slowly run your finger over the area of these known lentigines, you would not be able to feel them. They come in all sizes and, since they are the result of chronic sun exposure, are most prevalent in sun-exposed areas like the face, hands, and V of the neck.

We like to treat lentigines with liquid nitrogen, a treatment discussed in Chapter Seven. We apply frozen copper disks directly to the dark lentigo for two or three seconds. It is also possible to apply the liquid nitrogen by spraying or with Q-Tips™. The freezing causes a slight burning sensation for a minute or two. Over the next day, a scab usually forms, which may last from four to seven days. When the scab comes off, the dark spot looks the same as it did before or perhaps a little redder. It appears that the liquid nitrogen works by stopping the pigment cells from making excess pigment. At the time of freezing, the pigment is at the basal layer of the skin. It takes about four weeks to work its way up to the surface and out of the skin, at which time the spot disappears. We usually treat four or five lentigines in the first sessions. Then, if they fade satisfactorily, we treat the others four weeks later.

Liquid nitrogen works well for most patients, but there are other ways to treat lentigines, such as a bleach cream alone or in conjunction with trichloroacetic acid (TCA). If both are used, the lentigines are first treated with a 10 to 15 percent TCA solution. The area turns white and, in a day or two the whiteness is gone. At that time, bleach cream is started, applied twice a day. It is mandatory at this point to use a sunscreen at all times, because any exposure to ultraviolet light will stimulate the skin to make more pigment. The treatment may be repeated every three or four weeks until the results are satisfactory. Bleach creams used alone are discussed later in this chapter.

While we will not attempt to draw conclusions, we cannot resist observing that while our female patients see liver spots as a highly distasteful sign of aging, our male patients seldom ask to have them treated. Oh yes. Liver spots have nothing to do with the liver.

CHLOASMA AND MELASMA

Chloasma, the "mask of pregnancy," and melasma, a similar discoloration of the face seen most commonly in women who are taking oral contraceptives, can be treated with chemical peels. The tan and brown areas on the face, completely flat and smooth to the touch, are due to an increase in the size of the melanosomes, those pigment-containing granules produced in the melanocyte. When the melanosomes increase in size, they disperse throughout the higher levels of the epidermis, where they can be amenable to peels. If the pigment drops into the upper dermis, which it occasionally does, a superficial peel is of little use.

Since both are brought on by a change in the body's hormonal balance combined with exposure to ultraviolet light, hormone intake and exposure to the sun must be limited as much as possible. That means using a sunscreen that blocks both types of ultraviolet light—UVA and UVB. A bleach cream may also be used.

FRECKLES

Because freckles are not really a sign of aging, we mention them only briefly. Some of the treatments for aging skin also affect freckles. Chemical peels will reduce or remove them. Bleach creams have little effect.

BLEACH CREAMS

Bleach creams do not really bleach. Instead, they cause the skin to produce less pigment. Over the years, all sorts of substances have been used to bleach the skin including lemon juice, citric acid, tea (tannic acid), and salicylic acid. Ammoniated mercury in a 1 to 5 percent ointment was a commonly used bleach cream until mercury was banned in many countries. (It was sold over the counter, in fact; problems include contact sensitivity, discoloration, and kidney damage.)

Hydroquinone is currently the best lightening agent we know of. It was first used as a bleach cream in the late thirties, when rubber industry workers started developing areas of depigmentation from exposure to monobenzyl ether of hydroquinone. Monobenzyl ether of hydroquinone—still on the market as a bleach cream—was unpredictable. It could leave you with irregular, spotty depigmentation not only where the cream was applied but anywhere on the body. With hydroquinone as now used, pigmentation change occurs only where it is supposed to, i.e. where the cream is applied.

Such products as Eldoquin™, Eldoquin Forte™, Esoterica™, Astra™, or Melanax™ make hydroquinone available in different concentrations, most commonly 2, 3, and 4 percent. Hydroquinone can be used alone in a cream or lotion or in combination with other substances to enhance its effectiveness. The addition of sunscreens, for example, allows the hydroquinone to do its job while keeping out the ultraviolet light that stimulates production of pigment. The "Kligman formula"—hydroquinone, cortisone, and Vitamin A acid (the last a common acne preparation)—has become very popular. Salicylic acid added to hydroquinone will also enhance its effectiveness. We have been particularly pleased with a prescription medication called

Melanax®: its 3 percent hydroquinone in a special solution penetrates the skin quite well enabling more hydroquinone to reach the desired area.

Before using any hydroquinone solution, it's a good idea to perform an open patch test and make sure you are not allergic. Apply a small amount of the solution to a part of the body that does not get sun and where, if a reaction does occur, no one will notice. We suggest the inside of the arm. Rub a small amount on the spot twice a day for three days. If at the end of three days there is no reaction, go ahead and use the solution. Mild irritation occasionally results with any of these preparations but can be controlled with a 1 percent hydrocortisone cream.

Keep in mind that bleach creams are not wonder drugs. Getting an area to lighten after four to six weeks of treatment is considered a success. The result must then be maintained with a plain hydroquinone preparation and a sunscreen.

CORRECT USE OF A BLEACH CREAM

1.–Minimize sun exposure.

2.–Wear protective clothing.

3.–Use a broad-spectrum sunscreen (UVA and UVB) liberally.

4.–Keep bleach cream out of the eyes.

5.–Keep in mind that the safety of topical hydroquinone during pregnancy has not been established.

6.–If irritation occurs, and it cannot be controlled with the 1 percent hydrocortisone cream, stop treatment and see a physician.

7.–Be patient. They don't work overnight.

SKIN CANCER

This book would not be complete without a brief mention of skin cancer. With more people spending more time in the sun and wearing less clothing, we can expect skin cancer to reach epidemic proportions in the next decade. According to the Skin Cancer Foundation, if the incidence continues to increase at its present rate, over 5 million Americans will have a skin cancer diagnosed, and 90 percent of those skin cancers will be on parts of the body exposed to sunlight. Because people let skin cancer get out of hand, hundreds of thousands will be disfigured through scarring. A small number of them will lose all or part of their noses, eyes, lips, or ears. Fifty thousand will die.

What is the answer? As with any cancer, it has a lot to do with early detection. Detection, in turn, has a lot to do with public awareness and our knowledge of the problem. Since one out of every seven Americans will develop some form of skin cancer at some time in their lives, it is clear that we need to know more. At present, all we can talk about are connections, but the connections are very strong —between skin cancer and exposure to the sun and between skin cancer and exposure to chemicals such as arsenic. The sun plays a role in 90 percent of all skin cancer where the cause is known. Skin cancer appears in sun-damaged skin, but the lesions may have sent out roots known as "silent extensions" before they became visible on the surface.

Basal cell carcinoma is the most common form of skin cancer. It develops, as the name implies, from the basal layer of the skin. (The basal layer is the bottom layer of the epidermis and the epidermis is the uppermost layer of the skin.) It usually begins as a smooth, translucent, waxy growth, or papule, that can vary from pale yellow to pearl gray in color. Often it has a little blood vessel inside. Ninety percent of all cases appear on the face, most frequently in the fair-skinned. Since there are various types of basal cell carcinomas, it is important that a physician examine any suspected lesion at an early stage. Basal cell carcinomas may be pigmented or nonpigmented, scarlike, thick, hard, and/or ulcerated. Superficial basal cell carcinoma or multicentric carcinoma can look like psoriasis. If detected and treated early, basal cell carcinoma is curable.

Squamous cell carcinoma also occur primarily in sun-damaged areas of the body. Since they arise from the layer of cells directly above the basal level, where the cells grow faster, they are more aggressive than basal cell carcinoma. The tumors are usually shallow with hard borders. The base is red and granular and is covered by a crusted surface. They may occur in mucous membranes, scars (especially burn scars), and areas of previous radiation damage. Again, the secret to successful treatment is early detection.

Malignant melanoma is by far the most dangerous and life-threatening form of skin cancer. It accounts for two-thirds of all the skin cancer deaths reported. The latest information blames most cases on—you guessed it—the sun. What does it look like? The lesions are usually black or dark though they sometimes appear with no pigment at all. The torso, hands, feet, and face are the usual hosts. With time, it can change color, grow, itch, bleed, and/or give off a discharge. No carcinoma spreads more quickly throughout the body than melanoma, but new statistics have begun to show that, if detected *very* early, melanoma can also be curable.

There are many ways to treat skin cancer, including surgery, electrodessication and curettage, irradiation, and chemotherapy. Once a physician has made the diagnoses and identified the tumor, he can suggest the best form of therapy.

BASAL CELL AND
SQUAMOUS CELL CARCINOMA

1.–A new growth appears.

2.–An old growth begins to change character in any of the following ways:

Color—turns brown or red;

Size—grows larger;

Surface—crusts, scabs, erodes, or bleeds;

Symptoms—may itch or hurt and does not heal but, rather, gets larger.

MALIGNANT MELANOMA

1.–A new tan, brown, or black blemish appears.

2.–An old mole or "beauty mark" begins to change character in any of the following ways:

Color—gets darker or variable in color;

Size—gets larger or irregular in outline;

Surface—roughens, scales, erodes, or bleeds;

Symptoms—itches or hurts.

Source: Skin Cancer Foundation, New York.

QUESTIONS AND ANSWERS

Q. I have an important engagement this evening. If I have these facial blood vessels treated now, will I be presentable by tonight?

A. Yes. Most people have no noticeable side effects—except, of course, reduction or elimination of the blood vessels treated. In rare instances, small, hardly noticeable scabs form at the treatment site.

Q. A friend of mine had a dilated blood vessel on her cheek coagulated and now has an indentation at the site. Is this common?

A. This is a known side effect and must be taken into consideration, but it is very rare. We have treated thousands of blood vessels and have seen it occur only once. With time, it will often return to normal. If it persists, it can be elevated with injectable collagen. But we emphasize it is *very* rare.

Q. Can dilated blood vessels around the base of the nose be treated?

A. In that area, they tend to be a little larger, so the success rate is not as high as with finer, more superficial vessels. In addition the area is more sensitive and thus involves a little more pain.

Q. If you treat a blood vessel on my face, is it gone forever?

A. By treating the blood vessel, we do not eliminate the reason it dilated in the first place, nor have we stopped the on-going process. Therefore, a certain percentage of them will re-open and others can form in other places. The only solution is to treat them again.

Q. Do these red spots on my body have anything to do with something in my diet?

A. No, they are most likely dilated blood vessels, not related to diet. They are not dangerous; the only problem with them is cosmetic. Let us re-emphasize at this time that it's not a good idea to be your own doctor. If you have a new growth, let a physician examine it. Once you know what it is, you can make your own diagnosis if it recurs.

Q. Is there anything special I have to do for my liver spots after you treat them?

A. Once they are frozen, you can forget about them, even when they form scabs for a short time. You can get the scabs wet, cover them with makeup, whatever, without interfering with the treatment.

Q. What about these advertisements about fading "age spots"?

A. If they contain hydroquinone, they might work. A 4 percent hydroquinone preparation is better than a 2 percent preparation. It's a slow process and does not work for everyone. If you use such a preparation, you must use a broad-spectrum sunscreen along with it. We think light cryotherapy works better.

Q. Is skin cancer hereditary?

A. It is not hereditary *per se,* but the factors that make you susceptible to it are hereditary. Your skin type determines how much protection you will have from the sun. Your parents may also have something to do with your lifestyle and where you live and whether you develop the habit of spending much time outdoors.

Appendix:
How to Read a Cosmetics Label

Food and Drug Administration regulations define cosmetics as topical agents such as powders, creams, and lotions that affect personal grooming and appearance. They do not act upon the structure or function of the skin. Any product that clearly has an active agent is classified as a drug and is subject to review panels, testing, and generally more rigid controls. Cosmetics must state, on the package or an insert, their ingredients, listed in order of decreasing percentage. There is just one problem. The list of ingredients is Greek not only to the consumer but to many physicians. It takes a sophisticated chemist to truly make sense out of a cosmetics label.

In order to provide some kind of guide to these ingredients, we went down to the local cosmetics counter, picked up a dozen cosmetics at random, compiled a list of ingredients, and put them together in this appendix with an explanation of what they are, what they are used for, and their sensitivity potential. This is not meant to be, nor does it pretend to be, a complete dictionary of cosmetics. Such dictionaries are available and in paperback.

Our list includes a number of exotic ingredients, such as avocado oil and camomile, that have never really been tested scientifically but which have been in use for hundreds of years. We have included some of the claims made for such ingredients and, to distinguish the opinion of cosmetologists from scientific gospel, have placed such claims in quotation marks.

Whether or not an ingredient is "comedogenic" is based on the rabbit's ear test. Such ingredients are tested by applying them to a rabbit's ear for two weeks. Rabbit's ears form blackheads and clogged pores very easily. Non-comedogenic is not the same thing as "oil-free." There are a few oil-free products that do, in fact, cause blackheads on the rabbit's ear.

Allergic reaction from cosmetics is always a possibility. Those who are allergic to fragrances should know that some products labeled "unscented" do in fact have a small amount of fragrance to cover up the disagreeable smell of fatty acids and other ingredients.

Acacia—gum arabic, colorless, tasteless, used in cosmetics as thickener; vegetable gum and common sensitizer.

Acetic acid—clear, colorless solvent; vinegar is approximately 5 percent acetic acid; used in bleaching creams; mild irritant.

Acetol—see *lanolin*.

Acetyl—name given to acetic acid when combined with other substances.

Acid—solution with pH less than 7; releases hydrogen ions when dissolved in water.

Alcohol—fermentation product used as solvent; clear and colorless, very drying; external antiseptic.

Aliphatic—an oil; "fatty" series of hydrocarbons.

Allantoin—prepared from uric acid, used in many cosmetics for its "healing" qualities.

Almond oil—emollient; natural vegetable oil.

Almond paste—made from dried seeds of sweet almond; used as a cleanser.

Aloe vera—clear, viscous fluid from aloe plant leaf; 99 percent water with small amounts of amino acid and carbohydrates; added to many cosmetics for its "soothing" and "softening" effects.

Aluminum stearate—used for coloring and thickening in cosmetics.

Ambergris—fixative in fragrances obtained from sperm whale; 80 percent cholesterol.

Ammonium laureth sulfate—see *sodium lauryl sulfate.*

Amphoteric—capable of acting as either an acid or a base; used as surface active agents in detergents.

Antioxidant—inhibits oxidation, which prevents oils or fats from turning rancid, e.g. Vitamin C and E.

Aromatic—a chemical with an aroma.

Ascorbic acid—Vitamin C. Preservative and antioxidant in cosmetic creams and lotions.

Ascorbyl palmate—preservative and antioxidant used in cosmetics to prevent rancidity; derived from ascorbic acid.

Avocado oil—used in masks, shampoos; lubricating oil; contains natural vitamins.

Azulene—distilled from camomile flowers. Blue hydrocarbon used in cosmetics for aroma (camomile) and coloring; "anti-inflammatory" and "soothing."

Balsams (Peru, Mecca, Tola)—secreted from bruised plant (similar to resin); odor of vanilla or cinnamon; used in masks, perfumes, cream rinses; mildly irritating, may be sensitizing.

Beeswax—produced by bees in the making of the honeycomb; used in many cosmetics; emulsifier; creates heavier or "cushiony" feel.

Bentonite—purified clay; used in masks, as thickener and emulsifier.

Benzocaine—local anesthetic, can cause allergic dermatitis.

Benzophenone—sunblock agent both UVA and UVB; added to many cosmetics.

Benzyl alcohol—solvent, from plants, can be skin irritant.

Bergamot (oil of)—plant extract used in perfumes; common cause of photodermatitis.

Betaine—occurs in vegetables, used in resins.

BHA—butylated hydroxyanisole, preservative and antioxidant; can cause allergic reactions.

BHT—butylated hydroxytoluene; see *BHA* (similar).

Bismuth compounds—bismuth (metallic element) compounds used to give a pearl-colored frost or shine; can be sensitizing.

Borates (borax, boric acid)—antiseptic preservative or texturizer; cleansing properties; can be dangerous if ingested.

2 Bromo-2-Nitropropane 1, 3 diol—Bronopol®, used in manufacture of cosmetics and as propellant solvent; vapors can be irritating to mucous membranes.

Butyl (stearate)—a four-carbon hydrocarbon, from mineral oil; comedogenic, e.g. butyl stearate (emulsifier).

Butylene glycol—liquid humectant; comedogenic.

Butylparaben—most widely used preservative; see *parabens*.

Calcium pantothenate—B-complex vitamin (B_5) with calcium (salt); high concentration in royal (queen bee) jelly; emollient.

Camomile—see *chamomile*.

Camphor—used in many cosmetics for cooling effect, probably secondary to its anesthetic properties; very aromatic; can be sensitizing.

Carbomer (tea, 940, etc.)—emulsifying agent; acidic; thickener—alters viscosity and aids in stability.

Carnuba wax—texturizer in cosmetics from the wax tree; brown-colored solid.

Carotene (beta)—yellow/red color of carrots, used as coloring agent; used in production of Vitamin A.

Castor oil—from castor bean; used in many cosmetics (lipstick, for example); soothing to skin; shiny film when dry.

Cellulose gum—from the cell wall of plants; alters viscosity and aids in emulsion and stability.

Ceteth (Nos. 1–30)—compounds from cetyl, lauryl, stearyl and oleyl alcohols with ethylene oxide; surface active agents in many detergents.

Cetyl alcohol—fatty alcohol, imparts a sticky feel; emulsion stabilizer and emollient; very low degree of comedogenicity; found in spermaceti.

Chamomile—herb, very aromatic, flower used in cosmetics as coloring agents (contains azulene) and for aroma; used for its "soothing" and "healing" qualities.

Cholesterol—used in cosmetics as emulsifier and lubricant.

Citric acid—widely used as preservative, keeps emulsions from separating and prevents color changes; from citrus fruit fermentation.

Cocamide—see *coconut oil*.

Cocoa butter—softens and lubricates; solid fat from cocoa plant that melts at skin temperature; potential sensitizer; comedogenic.

Coconut oil—saturated fat, semisolid, good cleanser, lathers; used in shampoos, soaps, and ointments; potential irritant.

Colors (D & C, FD & C)—capable of producing color in food, drug, or cosmetic; D & C means can be used only in drugs and cosmetics, FD & C means can be used in foods, drugs, and cosmetics; colors are certified safe by FDA.

Corn meal—from corn cobs, face and bath powders.

Cornstarch—used in powders, hydrophilic; "soothing," can be sensitizing.

Cresol—eye and hair preparations, antiseptic and disinfectant derived from coal tar and wood; ingestion or excessive absorption can be dangerous.

Cucumber extract—used for cooling effect and pleasant aroma; has mild skin bleaching properties; certain tropical cucumber juice can be irritant.

Cyclamates—(sodium and calcium) artificial sweeteners, used in certain cosmetics; 30–40 times sweeter than sugar.

Cystine—sulfur containing amino acid (result of hydrolysis or breakdown of proteins).

Dehydroacetic acid (DHA)—used in cosmetics for its antifungal and antibacterial qualities; weak acid.

Demulcent—mucilagenous or oily preparation used to soothe inflammation, e.g. gum acacia (mucous membranes) or aloe vera.

Dibromsalan (4, 5 Dibromosalicylanilide)—antibacterial added to soaps, creams, and lotions; photosensitizing potential.

Dibutyl—hydrocarbon (C_8H_{18}); from mineral oil.

Dilauryl thiodipropionate—anti-oxident, usually used to protect vegetable oils; preservative.

Dimethicone—silicone oil used topically as skin protector.

Dioctyl sodium sulfosuccinate—waxlike consistency, used as wetting agent in bubble bath, cleansing lotions, and to liquefy gums.

DMDM Hydantoin—(1, 3 dimethylol—5,5—dimethyl hydantoin) water soluble crystals that release formaldehyde preservative; hydantoin derived from allantoin.

EDTA—see *ethylenediamine tetraacetic acid.*

Emulsifier—agents that help in the production of emulsions, e.g. sulfated alcohols, stearates, polysorbates, PEGS, etc.

Emulsion—a homogeneous mixture of two or more nonmixable substances, e.g. oil and water.

Essence—that basic or most desirable properties, i.e. flavor or aroma, which remains in extracted substance.

Essential oils—liquid (oily) obtained from plants and retaining the basic properties (taste and smell); some also have germicidal, antiseptic, and/or preservative qualities.

Estrone—obtained from urine of pregnant women, mares

and human placenta; occasionally found in "hormone" creams or lotions; such small quantities are present that they are not biologically active.

Ethanol—ethyl alcohol, used as astringent, antiseptic.

Ethylenediamine tetraacetic acid—widely used preservative anti-oxidant by its ability to sequester trace metals.

Fatty acids—made up of carbon, hydrogen, and oxygen; saturated means no double bonds, i.e. maximum number of hydrogen; unsaturated means one or more double bonds, therefore fewer hydrogen ions; e.g. capric, lauric, myrisitic, oleic palmite and stearic.

Fatty alcohols—alcohols made from fatty acids used in creams and lotions, give silky feel, varying degree of comedogenicity.

F, D, & C Blue; F, D, & C Yellow; F, D, & C Red—see *colors.*

Fe oxides—iron oxide, color additive, red, brown, yellow, or black, depending on purity, water, and oxygen content.

Fragrance—pleasant aroma, scent, or odor; can be listed as such on cosmetic labels without further explanation.

Galvanic current—a direct and constant current used in producing chemical reactions.

Ginseng—Chinese herb, also grows in North America; added to cosmetics for aroma and "stimulant" properties.

Glutaral—amino acid used in emollients; aromatic.

Glycerin—humectant; can absorb moisture from the air; emollient.

Glyceryl stearate—humectant; very low degree comedogenicity.

Grape seed oil—used in lubricating creams; hypoallergenic.

Green soap—soap composed of linseed oil.

Humectant—wetting or moistening qualities; used to preserve water content in creams and lotions, e.g. glycerin, propylene glycol, etc.

Hydrocarbon—organic compound made up of hydrogen and carbon, e.g. petroleum, mineral oils, etc.

Hydrogenated—added hydrogen gas to liquid oils, e.g. hydrogenated lanolin; changes melting point so that liquid oils become semi-solid fats; also protects substance from breakdown due to oxidation.

Hydrolyzed animal protein—breakdown of collagen with water to form a simpler compound, i.e. smaller "particles."

Imidazolidinyl urea—see *urea*.

Isodecyl oleate—see *oleic acid*.

Isopropyl alcohol (IPA)—antibacterial, astringent, not for consumption.

Isopropyl myristate—myristate (sec) combined with fatty acid; aids absorption; comedogenic.

Jojoba oil—from jojoba bean; lubricating oil used in many cosmetics and hair products.

Kaolin—filler used to equalize the amount of pigment to the desired shade; blotting properties.

Keratin amino acids—protein obtained from hair, hoofs, horns, etc., used in hair products.

L. Cysteine—essential amino acid used in hair products and creams; may promote "wound healing."

Lactic acid—breakdown product of glucose, used in fresheners; higher concentrations are caustic to skin.

Laneth (5 through 40)—see *lanolin alcohol*.

Lanolin—from fleece of sheep (wool grease, wool wax, wool fat); natural substance used in cosmetics as humectant and emulsifier; very common sensitizer (allergan); comedogenic; listed under many names, e.g. amberlate P sterolan, acetol, acetulan, waxolan, lantrol, amerchol, langgene, etc.

Lanolin alcohol—solid waxy material derived from lanolin; emulsifier, emollient; comedogenic.

Lauric acid—component of vegetable fats, soaps and detergents; foam producing.

Lauryl alcohol—from coconut oil; used in detergents; has foaming properties.

Lauryl sulfate (sodium, zinc, calcium, etc.)—used in shampoos for degreasing ability and foaming properties; also emulsifier; comedogenic.

Lecithin—emollient and anti-oxidant; claimed to "stimulate" oil glands; found in egg yolk; emulsifier.

Linoleic acid—emulsifier; fatty acid found in vegetable oils.

Magnesium aluminum silicate—used as filler and coloring agent; mild astringent.

Menthol—from mint oils (peppermint) or synthetically from thymol; mild local anesthetic; aromatic; "cooling" effect on skin.

Mineral oil—used in many cosmetics; from liquid hydrocarbons; lubricant; leaves film on skin; certain preparations are comedogenic.

Musk (ambrette)—secretion from male musk deer used for its odor in perfumes and medicines; can cause photosensitive reaction.

Myristyl myristate—emollient; in animal and vegetable fats; used in shampoos, creams, and soaps.

NaCl—sodium chloride (salt); humectant when small amount added to emollient.

Nonoxynol (2-50)—surface active agent; emulsifier in hand creams.

Norvaline—protein amino acid.

Octyl dimethyl PABA—Ester of para-aminobenzoic acid used for sunscreening quality.

Oleic acid—unsaturated fatty acid from animal and/or vegetable fats and oils; used in creams, soaps, lipsticks, etc; mildly irritating.

Padimate-O—see *octyl dimethyl PABA.*

Panthenol—part of Vitamin B complex; used in hair products and emollients.

Paraben (methyl and propyl)—widely used preservatives; also antibacterial and antifungal; common sensitizer.

PEG—see *polyethylene glycol.*

Petrolatum (Vaseline®, petroleum jelly)—semisolid hydrocarbon from petroleum; used in many cosmetics; has "greasy" feel; comedogenic.

Placenta—an exotic additive to "remove" wrinkles; there is no evidence that it is effective.

Polyethylene glycol (PEG)—used in many products for its insulating properties, i.e. improves resistance to moisture.

Polyglyceryl—from edible vegetable fats and fatty acid esters; emulsifier.

Poly-sorbate (20–85)—emulsifier in creams and lotions; stabilizes essential oils; rarely sensitizing.

Potassium sorbate—preservative, especially against mold and yeast.

PPG (buteth, glycerol, etc.)—represents a polymer (group of substances) of different alcohols, ethylene oxide and propylene oxide; consistency of petrolatum yet is water soluble; lotions and hairdressings.

Pristane—hydrocarbon from shark liver and ambergris; lubricant.

Propylene glycol—humectant, solvent, and wetting agent; used in many cosmetics.

Pyridoxine HCl—Vitamin B_6; "soothing" to skin.

Quaternary ammonium compounds—used in many products as preservatives, antimicrobials, antiseptics and deodorizers, e.g. benzalkonium chloride.

Rose water—made by distilling fresh flowers, used as perfume.

Rosemary oil—from fresh rosemary flowers used in perfumes, liniments, and hair tonics.

Salicylic acid—added to cosmetics for its antimicrobial properties, also acts as keratolytic and skin softener.

Sesame oil—emollient, used in moisturizers, etc.

Sodium borate—preservative and emulsifier; can be irritant due to its drying effect.

Sodium dehydroacetate—a preservative; antimicrobial and antifungal in cosmetics.

Sodium lauryl sulfate—an excellent surfactant and degreaser; may be an irritant; comodogenic.

Sodium PCA—naturally occurring humectant in the skin (sodium pyrrolidone carboxylic acid).

Sorbitol—a humectant; velvety feel to skin; used in many cosmetics.

Soy glyceride—emollient, from soy bean, used in soaps, shampoos, and bath oils.

Spermaceti (synthetic)—base in many creams and ointments; from sperm whale; increases viscosity.

Squalene—unsaturated hydrocarbon from shark liver; surface active agent, used with hair dyes.

Stearic acid—fatty acid from animal fats and oils; many cosmetics, especially cream and soaps; gives pearl color and silky feel to creams; comedogenic.

Stearyl alcohol—prepared from sperm whale oil; adds texture to product; antifoam agent.

Sunflower seed oil—contains large amounts of Vitamin E; lubricant, used in soaps.

Surface-active agent—makes contact between skin and cosmetic easier, e.g. lecithin.

Surfactant—see *surface-active agent.*

Talc—powdered magnesium silicate, insoluble in water; coloring agent.

Titanium dioxide—white pigment used as an opacifier in sunscreens.

Tocopheryl acetate—Vitamin E; anti-oxidant in cosmetics.

Triclosan—broad-spectrum, antimicrobial agent added to soaps and creams.

Triethanolamine—made from ethyl oxide; hydrophilic; oil emulsifier.

Tween (20 and 80)—surfactants acting as a detergent; emulsifier; hydrophilic; comedogenic.

Urea—natural humectant secreted through sweat glands, used in many moisturizers.

Vegetable oil—obtained from plants, e.g. peanut, sesame,

olive, and cottonseed; used in many "hypoallergenic" cosmetics.

Wetting agent—water soluble substance that makes liquids spread easier or penetrate better; lowers surface tension.

Witchhazel extract—70–80 percent alcohol; astringent and anesthetic; skin freshener.

Zinc sulfate—zinc plus sulfuric acid; astringent.

Glossary

Acid balance—cosmetic term meaning that the pH of the product is the same as the pH of the skin or hair.

Acne surgery—includes removing comedones, incision, drainage of acne pustules, deep pore cleansing.

Acneiform—skin eruption that looks like acne (blackheads, whiteheads, papules, and/or pustules).

Actinic—from Greek god Aktis or ray, an adjective implying that ultraviolet light rays are a causative factor.

Actinic keratosis—red, scaling, often raised lesion, occurring in sun-exposed areas secondary to chronic sun exposure.

Acute—short or brief in duration; not chronic.

Adnexa—structures found in the skin; e.g. hair, nails, sweat, and oil glands.

Adulterate—to make a pure substance impure with additives, e.g. early "silicone" formulae.

Alkali—pH greater than 7, will neutralize acid, capable of making soaps from fats.

Allergen—any substance that can initiate an allergic reaction.

Allergic—reactive to certain substances resulting in skin eruption, hayfever, rhinitis, etc.

Alopecia—baldness.

Amino acid—building blocks of proteins.

Anesthetic—substance that decreases sensation of pain.

Angioma—a growth consisting of a collection of blood vessels (hemangioma).

Antibody—a substance produced by the immune system to react with and neutralize antigens.

Antigen—a substance considered foreign by the body that results in formation of antibodies, which in turn results in a disease state.

Antihistamine—medication used to negate the effect of histamine, a substance that can be released in the skin resulting in the itch sensation.

Antiseptic—agent used to produce asepsis (germ free state).

Arterioles—small ending of an artery, finally ending in a capillary.

Arthralgia—joint pains.

Aseptic—free from bacteria capable of causing infection as in aseptic technique.

Asteatosis—dry skin, especially when associated with lack of sebum.

Astringent—a clear liquid with a high percentage of alcohol, used to "refresh" the skin by its cooling action (evaporation).

Autoimmune disease—where the body forms antibodies to one or more of its own naturally occurring constituents.

Basal cell carcinoma (or epithelioma)—malignant growth of the cells of the basal layer of the epidermis.

Basal layer—bottom layer of the epidermis, closest to dermis; has ability to divide into two cells.

Basophilic degeneration—refers to staining characteristics of histochemical preparation (slide) with changes in the collagen (and elastin) from normal pink color to bluish; secondary to chronic UVL exposure.

Benign—mild, not malignant.

Blackhead—open comedone of acne; refers to plug in pilosebaceous opening.

Blusher—a powdered rouge used for contour shading.

Burn (first, second, and third degree)—injury to skin caused by heat, chemical, X-ray, friction, electricity, UVL, etc; first degree—redness and swelling; second degree—

redness, swelling and blisters; third degree—redness, swelling, loss of tissue.

Canities—gray or grayish white hair.

Capillary—smallest portion of blood vessels.

Carbolic acid—see *phenol*.

Carbon dioxide (CO₂)—result of combustion of carbon with air to result in carbonic acid gas.

Cardiotoxic—harmful to the heart.

Carotene—yellow-red color found in carrots, sweet spuds, yolk; colored lipoid hydrocarbons; too much in the blood can result in jaundice-like skin color *(carotenemia)*.

cc—cubic centimeter (see *milliliter*).

Centigrade scale—boiling is 100 degrees centigrade; freezing is 0 degrees centigrade.

Chloasma—irregular, mottled, relatively large areas of increased pigment on the face; also known as the "mask of pregnancy."

Chronic—taking place continually over a long time; opposite of acute.

Cicatrix—scar.

Coagulate/coagulation—to clot, as with blood.

Cold cream—cleansing cream (emulsion), combination of mineral oil, beeswax, borax, and water; as water evaporates, it "cools" the skin.

Collagen—from Greek word meaning "glue," fibrillar substance comprising the lion's share of the dermis.

Collagen-vascular disease—disease states involving collagen and blood vessels, e.g. lupus erythematosus.

Comedogenicity—ability to cause open and closed comedones ("blackheads" and "whiteheads") in susceptible people.

Comedone/comedo (open and closed)—the "plug" that obstructs the sebaceous gland duct (a whitehead is closed; a blackhead is open).

Contraindication—should not be done or used.

Corium—see *dermis*.

Cosmetic—substance used for adornment and beautification.

Cosmetician—a person professionally trained to use cosmetics.

Cosmetologist—dedicated and skilled in the art of "creating" and improving beauty.

Cryotherapy—treatment with contact application of a cold substance, e.g. liquid nitrogen (minus 196 degrees centigrade).

Cubic centimeter (cc)—Equal to one milliliter (a thousandth of a liter) in metric system of fluid capacity.

Curettage—scraping away tissue with a curette.

Curette—instrument with circular hollow end, the edge of the circle being sharpened, and a long handle.

Cutaneous horn—compacted keratin that looks and feels like a horn *(cornu cutaneum)*.

Cutis—see *dermis*.

Dermabrasion—removal of skin by mechanical means with a revolving wire brush, fraise, or sandpaper.

Dermis—"true skin" layer below the epidermis and above the subcutaneous fat; made up of collagen, elastin, and connective tissue.

Desquamation—peeling off of scales, either naturally or by mechanical/chemical means.

Dessicate—to dry out.

Detergent—cleansing agent like soap except that it is made from chemicals, not natural fats.

Dry ice—solid carbon dioxide.

Ecchymosis—large leakage of blood into a tissue space with resultant purple color.

Edema—accumulation of water, lymph, or serum proteins that results in swelling of an area.

Elastic fibers—found in dermis; keep skin from stretching too far and help it return to normal contour.

Electrodessication—drying out of tissue using electrosurgical procedure to burn tissue.

Embolism—a substance that results in the plugging of a blood vessel.

Emollient—an externally applied material to prevent or counteract the symptoms of dryness; oil plus water plus emulsifying agent.

Emulsion—the homogeneous mixture of two substances that do not normally dissolve in each other, with an added emulsifier.

Ephilis—freckle.

Epidermabrasion—removal of residual scales of outermost layer of epidermis by mild abrasion.

Epidermis—outermost layer of skin, multilayered; ranges from the basal layer, next to the dermis, to the stratum corneum, which is on the surface.

Epithelium—cellular lining on the surface of the body, i.e. epidermis.

Erythema—redness.

Erythemogenic—ability to produce redness, e.g. UVL rays of correct wavelength.

Eschar—scab or crust usually secondary to a heat or chemical burn.

Esthetician—a professionally trained person dedicated to the art and beauty of the skin.

Fahrenheit scale—water freezes at 32 degrees Fahrenheit and boils at 212 degrees Fahrenheit.

Farmer's and sailor's skin—skin ravaged by years of sun, wind, heat, and cold.

Fatty acid—saturated hydrocarbon chains used to make soap and detergents, e.g. stearic, lauric, or myristic acid used in many cosmetics.

Fibroblast—cells in dermis that produce collagen.

5-Fluorouracil—an anticancer drug used externally to treat sun-damaged skin and solar keratoses.

Glabella—the area on the face between the eyebrows.

Glycerin—a strongly hydrophilic substance, used as an emollient or humectant.

Hemangioma—see *angioma.*

Hematoma—discolored, enlarged, or swollen area secondary to leakage of blood into tissue.

Hirsute—hairy, usually excessively.

Hives—see *urticaria.*

Hormone—a substance formed in an organ in one part of the body and transplanted via the blood stream to have an effect on another organ.

Humectant—a substance that aids in retaining water in the skin.

Hydrophilic—a "water-attracting" or "water-holding" substance.

Hygroscopic—refers to ability to absorb and retain water.

Hyperpigmentation—excessive coloration.

Hypertrophy—enlarged to greater than normal size or number.

Hypodermal—area immediately below the dermis.

Hypopigmentation—area of decreased skin coloration.

Immune—Unresponsive to or protected from a certain disease state or failing to benefit.

Induration/indurated—physical hardness.

Isopropyl alcohol (IPA)—70 percent alcohol derived from propylene, used as disinfectant and in some cosmetics.

Jowl—lax skin hanging from jaw or cheeks, as a "double chin."

Keloid—an enlarged scar, a result of overexuberant healing where the scar is larger than the original injury.

Keratin—protein material that makes up stratum corneum, hair, and nails.

Keratolysis—dissolution or separation of keratin.

Keratosis—disruption of growth of the outer layer of the stratum corneum; different types look and act differently; usually preceded by an adjective, e.g. actinic keratosis.

Lentigine—lentil-shaped dark spot, secondary to chronic UVL exposure.

Lentigo—see *lentigine.*

Lesion (primary)—first change in the skin grossly recognizable secondary to disease state, hurt, or injury.

Lidocaine—see *Xylocaine* ®.

Liver spot—dark spot secondary to chronic UVL most commonly on backs of hands and face; not related to liver.

Lotion—liquid solution.

Lymph—clear fluid of the lymphatic system (tied in to the body's immune mechanism).

Lymphangioma—excess development of lymph vessels resulting in raised, clear lesion.

Macule—blemish or dark mark that is flat, i.e. not raised above skin surface.

Malignant—any rapidly developing problem with a bad conclusion (usually refers to cancer).

Melanin—colored protein complex formed in pigment-making cells, e.g. the melanocyte.

Melanocyte—a cell that produces melanin, found in basal layer of epidermis, and responsible for skin color.

Melanosome—organelle within melanocyte that contains melanin.

Melasma—see *chloasma* (same problem, but not related to pregnancy).

Milliliter (ml)—one thousandth of a liter or approximately 0.034 fluid ounces.

ml—see *milliliter.*

Morphology—having to do with structure or form, i.e. what something looks like.

Myalgia—muscle pain.

Nanometer—one billionth of a meter; used to measure wavelength of electromagnetic radiation (UVL).

Naso-labial fold—wrinkle lines starting at the side of the nose and running down around mouth (grin lines).

Nephrotoxic—damaging to the kidney.

Nevus, nevi—lesion made of collection of pigment cells, commonly referred to as moles.

Ostium—opening of pilosebaceous unit onto skin (also referred to as a pore).

Ounce (oz)—one sixteenth of a pound, 30 grams, or 30 ml.

Pathogenic—capable of causing disease.

Percutaneous—ability to penetrate through the skin.

pH—the degree of acidity (pH less than 7) or alkalinity (pH greater than 7); pH 2 is more acidic than pH 5.

Phenol—carbolic acid, made from coal tar, used in face peels and as disinfectant and anesthetic; fatal poisoning can occur via skin absorption.

Photoallergic—interactive of light plus some substance on the skin or taken internally that results in skin eruption.

Photosensitivity—excessive sensitivity to light or reaction of light (sun) plus an internal or topically applied medicine resulting in skin rash.

Phototoxic—interaction of light plus some substance on skin to result in an irritancy type skin reaction.

Pilosebaceous unit—refers to the close interaction of the hair follicle and sebaceous (oil) gland; the sebaceous gland duct empties into the hair follicle before exiting onto the skin.

Pore—opening or passageway, e.g., sweat duct onto skin (see *ostium*).

Post-op—time directly after an operation.

Proteolytic—a substance (organic) capable of breaking protein down to its constituent parts.

Pruritis—itching.

Purpura—bleeding under the skin, usually macular; purple color.

Re-epithelization—growth that results in correcting a defect in the epithelium.

Resorcinol—used in many cosmetics, obtained from resins;

antiseptic, preservational, astringent, and anti-itch actions.

Rosacea—chronic redness on central part of face (cheeks and nose), often with telangiectasia and acneiform lesions.

Salicylic acid—made from phenol plus carbon dioxide; used in many cosmetics, e.g. anti-itch, antiseptic, keratolytic, preservative.

Sebaceous gland—produces sebum; associated with hair follicles.

Sebum—only material produced by sebaceous gland; mixture of fatty acids, triglycerides, phosphatides, waxes, and alcohols.

Silicon—nonmetallic tetrad element containing silica (Si).

Silicone—organic compound made of silicon, oxygen, and methane (dimethyl polysiloxanes)

Solar elastosis—abnormal elastic fibers, as visualized through the microscope, UVL induced.

Spider—see *telangiectasia.*

Squamous cell carcinoma—skin cancer originating from the squamous layer of the epidermis (layer above basal layer).

Stratum corneum—outermost layer of epidermis, made up of dead cells (fibrous protein).

Subacute—not chronic, not acute.

Subcutaneous—directly under the skin.

Substantivity—the ability of sunscreens to remain effective through swimming and sweating.

Superficial—shallow, on the surface, not deep.

Surface tension—the measure of imbalance of molecular forces on or near a surface.

Surfactant—a surface-active substance that can bind to both water and oil; when added to an oil-water mixture aids emulsification, e.g. soap.

Systemic—widespread throughout the body.

TCA—see *trichloroacetic acid.*

Telangiectasia—small blood vessels, often a dilated capillary; if it has small red offshoots, is sometimes referred to as "spiders."

Thymol iodide powder—antibacterial powder often used after face peels.

Toxic—refers to poison or toxin.

Trauma—wound or injury.

Trichloroacetic acid—caustic; used in acid face peels.

Tumor—swelling or growth; does *not* imply malignancy.

Urticaria—hives or wheals.

UVA, UVB, UVC—arbitrary designations for certain wavelengths of the electromagnetic wavelength spectrum (ultraviolet to infrared); UVA is 320–400 nanometers; UVB is 280–320; UVC is 200–280.

Vital signs—measure of certain parameters necessary for life to exist, e.g. blood pressure, temperature, heart rate and rhythm, respiration, etc.

Welt—wheal, usually linear.

Xeroderma—dry skin.

Xylocaine® / lidocaine—a local, injectible anesthetic.

Zyderm™ Collagen Implant—injectible bovine collagen.

Index

(For additional listings, check the Glossary)